Managing
Your Mind
and Mood
Through Food

Also by Judith J. Wurtman, Ph.D.:

EATING YOUR WAY THROUGH LIFE
THE CARBOHYDRATE CRAVER'S DIET

Managing Your Mind and Mood Through Food

Judith J. Wurtman, Ph.D.
with
Margaret Danbrot

Harper & Row, Publishers, New York
Cambridge, Philadelphia, San Francisco, Washington
London, Mexico City, São Paulo, Singapore, Sydney

First PERENNIAL LIBRARY edition published 1988.

Library of Congress Cataloging-in-Publication Data

Wurtman, Judith J.
  Managing your mind and mood through food.

  Bibliography: p.
  Includes index.
  1. Nutrition—Psychological aspects. 2. Mood (Psychology) I. Danbrot, Margaret.
II. Title.
[QP141.W87 1988]   613.2   87-45676
ISBN 0-06-097138-X (pbk.)

93 94 95 MPC 10 9 8 7

To the memory of my father,
Alexander Hirschhorn,
and my mother-in-law and father-in-law,
Hilda and Samuel Wurtman

Contents

ACKNOWLEDGMENTS   ix

1. The Food / Mind / Mood Connection   3
2. Food / Mind / Mood Strategies—They're Safe   13
3. Food, Mood, and the Brain   17
4. Testing Your Food / Mind / Mood Response   33
5. All-Day, Everyday Power Eating   55
6. Caffeine: A Mind- and Mood-Boosting Plus   95
7. Meals That Really Work at Work   107
8. Preperformance Meals:
    Eating for a Winning Presentation   121
9. Conference-Goers' Guide
    to High-Achievement Eating   145
10. Conference Planners' Confidential   171
11. How to Eat to Beat Your Inner Clock   187
12. Travelers' Advisory: Anti–Jet Lag Tactics for
    Better Business and Pleasure Trips   207
13. Eating to Ease Stress   229
14. Food / Mind / Mood and Your Future   247

APPENDIX A   Stress-Easing, Mind-Focusing,
             Sleep-Inducing High-Carb Snacks   251
APPENDIX B   Sample Recipes for Recommended
             Dishes   255
BIBLIOGRAPHY   265
INDEX   267

Acknowledgments

This book would not have been written without the support and efforts of many people. The first is my husband, Richard, who urged me to consider writing such a book and, once I had made the decision to do so, successfully protected me against competing demands on my time so that it could be written. I am especially grateful for his efforts in making sure that I had both privacy and the word processor whenever I needed them.

This book also owes its existence to Helen Rees, my agent, who responded to my tentative and vague ideas for this book with such enthusiasm that I began to believe it could be done. She was always available to solve any problem, to listen to my complaints, and to relieve the tedium of writing with her witty and wise phone calls.

Of course, the major contributor to this book's existence is my coauthor, Margaret Danbrot. Her uncanny ability to translate ideas into easily understood and immensely readable concepts, her incredible good humor under enormous pressure, and her patience in handling seemingly endless revisions made working with her an absolute delight.

My publisher, Eleanor Rawson, must receive my special thanks. She taught me how to inform the nonscientist about what we do and its relevance, and I am grateful for her insistence on complete and thorough scientific explanations throughout the book.

I must also mention those individuals whose scientific contributions made this book possible. The research carried out by my colleagues—notably, Dr. Bonnie Spring, Dr. Harris Lieberman, and Dr. Norman Rosenthal—and many others has pushed the idea that food can affect the mind and mood out of the realm of old wives' tales and into the area of normative science. Their research demanded not only creativity and labor but courage to investigate concepts that no one thought could be tested in a laboratory situation. The results of their research have had an impact on all of our lives.

My gratitude also goes to my associates at M.I.T.—Sharon Reynolds, Rita Tsay, Gail Garfield, Ann Lee, Elizabeth Keane—and the many others at the M.I.T. Clinical Research Center whose extraordinary competence made our research on nutrients and their effect on behavior possible.

Finally, I have to thank Wolfgang Amadeus Mozart, whose music was always there to sustain me throughout the writing of this book.

Managing Your Mind and Mood Through Food

1. The Food/Mind/Mood Connection

Do you want a more alert, more focused, more *productive* mind?

Do you want to be able to calm down, unwind, and relax at will . . . even get to sleep on demand?

Do you want to ease feelings of stress or anxiety and enhance your overall sense of well-being?

Whether you are striving for personal or professional excellence or both, I'm going to assume that your answer to all of the questions above is an enthusiastic, unqualified *yes*! And in the chapters that follow I will tell you everything you need to know to achieve all of these benefits, and more.

As a research scientist at M.I.T., as well as in my private practice, I have helped thousands of people to maximize their performance, power their brains, and manage their moods. The simple, proven techniques that have changed their lives for the better can do the same for you.

You will learn how food can help you bounce back when mental lethargy or a loss of enthusiasm dampens your ability to get things done, and how to compose yourself when edginess or distractibility threatens to interfere at work, at play, or in your relationships with others.

You will learn how food can help you focus your mind when the situation calls for clear thinking and creative problem-solving—and how to quicken your responses when speed is of the essence.

You will learn how food can help you ward off "brain fatigue" so you can stay up late to finish a report or study for an exam, and still perform at your peak the following morning. You will also learn how *the right food* can help you deal with the feelings of frustration and anxiety that lead to overeating and weight gain!

In short, you will learn how to use food to shift at will from a state of mind that works against you into one that works for you! And you can learn to make these mood changes occur almost instantly, without investing in long hours of therapy and without drugs—in fact, with practically no effort on your part other than following the easy-to-use guidelines in this book.

You already know from personal experience that whether you are up or down, calm or agitated, focused or distracted, the way you feel can make all the difference in how successfully you work, study, create, play, and interact with others.

But you may not have been aware of how many of the foods you eat affect those moods and behaviors. Though the results of studies linking food intake to mood and behavior—projects carried out at M.I.T., at the Harvard Medical School, at the National Institutes of Health, and at other prestigeous research centers—have appeared in many of the specialized scientific publications and medical journals, little of this information has been widely reported in the popular press.

Nevertheless, research done by my colleagues and me at M.I.T. and elsewhere confirms that certain foods have a number of previously unsuspected capabilities.

Simply put, some foods influence the production and function of chemicals in the brain that are directly involved in determining mood, mental energy, performance, and behavior. Some foods increase mental alertness, speed, and accuracy and will tend to make you feel more motivated and energetic. But these same foods, eaten under different circumstances, can also produce feelings of tension and irritability. Other foods are natural tranquilizers that calm feelings of anxiety and stress. However, depending on certain factors, such as the time of day when they are eaten, these foods can also make you feel slowed-down, sluggish, even sleepy.

Further, mental states can be modified—usually within half an hour or less—when an "antidote" food is eaten. For example, a calming food will counter a hyper, nervous, or anxious state. An energizing food will offset "brain drain" and sleepiness.

What makes all of these new findings so significant is that the foods capable of producing these remarkable mood and behavior changes are *not* little-known, rarely encountered exotica. They are the normal, ordinary foods most of us enjoy every single day of our lives and can easily find in our supermarkets.

In my work as a researcher in many of the food/mind/mood studies, and as a nutritional counselor with my own private practice, I have been in a unique position to test and retest the new theories, both in the lab and with real-life people in real-life situations. I was able to take the results of my laboratory work at the M.I.T. Clinical Research Center and immediately use them, when applicable, with private clients. Feedback from clients often inspired my colleagues at M.I.T. and me to move into new areas of investigation, and the results of these new experiments could then be reconfirmed with clients.

This shuttling back and forth between lab, clinical work, and private practice—comparing scientific data with the responses from patients and clients—allowed me to develop and then fine-tune dozens of simple, practical, and effective applications for the new food/mind/mood findings.

From the beginning I was convinced that the research we were doing was important and would have many exciting, even revolutionary implications. But even I didn't anticipate how useful it would turn out to be.

For example, in working with clients, I discovered that the creative ones who frequently claimed they could do original thinking only at certain times of day suddenly were able to "work smart" whenever they wanted to if they adhered to our suggestions for meals and snacks. Business people were able to maintain that all-important competitive edge if they ate according to these instructions. Academics and other professionals, as well as people in managerial and sales positions, found that by applying these food guidelines they were able to withstand the rigors of all-day conferences and meetings—and continue to function in top form for hours on end, even as colleagues wilted. Travelers who followed these guidelines were able to reach their destinations fresher and more alert, ready to work or play immediately on arrival. And long-distance travelers reported feeling little or no jet lag!

In applying the basic food/mind/mood findings, as revealed by research carried out at hundreds of scientific institutions here and abroad, to more and more of the people who came to us for nutritional counseling, one thing became increasingly clear: The range of big and little problems that can be alleviated simply by eating the right food at the right time is practically limitless!

Food, Mind, Mood, and *You*

Right now, at this very moment, for better or for worse, the food you ate at your last meal or snack is affecting your mood and behavior. (I hope it's helping you absorb and retain what you're reading!) Depending on when, what, and how much you ate, the effect may be subtle or pronounced, but it's *there*.

The meals and snacks you eat later on will affect the way you feel afterward. Whether you are groggy, sharp, tense, or composed, food will be a major factor.

In the past, whether food worked for you or against you usually was a matter of luck or chance. It no longer has to be that way. With all that we now know about the food/mind/ mood connection and how to apply related basic principles, you can begin to select the breakfasts, lunches, dinners, and snacks that will power your brain, modify your moods, and in the process make you a more effective, motivated, and perhaps even more *contented* individual.

In the next few chapters, I will show you how to eat to ensure that you function at your peak each day. And I will show you what to eat when you want to relax and reduce tension. And since some days are more demanding than others—professionally, emotionally, or both—I will give you special guidelines for special situations, including frustration, predeadline stress, and the inevitable crises at work or at home.

But before we move on to our food/mind/mood strategies and the details of why and how they can change your life, I would like to make a few points about the eating programs you will soon be sharing.

- *Food/mind/mood strategies won't "cure" you of anything.*

It is very important to make clear right here at the beginning that the principles and programs described throughout this book won't solve any serious physical or mental problems you may have. If you are in poor health, physically or mentally— for example, if you lack energy because of an underlying organic problem or if you are depressed or highly anxious—

eating the right food at the right time may help you feel a bit better, but that is not enough. You need professional, one-on-one help, and I urge you to get it if you are not already involved in treatment.

Food-mood strategies alone won't change bad habits, either. They won't miraculously make you give up cigarettes, quit biting your nails, or stop procrastinating. Nor will they lead automatically to a better job or a promotion or make you a winner at tennis or golf. We are not dealing with magic and wish fulfillment, but with hard science. With all that in mind, however, it is worth noting that by powering your brain, "upping" your mental energy, and giving you greater control over your moods, these strategies *will* increase your potential for success in *all* areas of your life.

• *Food/mind/mood strategies go beyond good nutrition.*

I am going to make the assumption here and throughout this book that your diet is reasonably well balanced—not necessarily textbook perfect, but at least adequate in terms of the nutrients it supplies. If your diet is less than adequate—if, for example, you do not get enough vitamins or you are suffering from an iron deficiency—you probably will continue to experience mental and physical fatigue no matter how faithfully you adhere to the food/mind/mood strategies.

I also want to emphasize that this is not just another book about good nutrition, although you will find nutritional suggestions sprinkled throughout. A good diet is important. But even a superior diet all by itself won't allow you to alter your moods at will. A superior diet alone won't enable you to increase your mental energy and efficiency instantly when the pressure is on, or to calm down and quiet your mind quickly when you want to relax. Only the food/mind/mood strategies that follow will do that.

Further, megavitamins and minerals and other dietary supplements play no role in these mind- and mood-modifying programs. If you are now taking extra vitamins and minerals and are convinced that they are beneficial and make you feel better, you may as well continue with them. (Just remember that megadoses of most supplements can be harmful!) Taking huge daily doses of vitamins and minerals over and above the amounts required to fulfill your body's needs *won't* power your brain and help you manage your moods.

But eating certain foods in a particular sequence at specific times *will*!

Food/Mind/Mood Strategies and Allergies

The food/mind/mood connection that we are concerned with in this book is a basic, normal, and universal phenomenon. Virtually every healthy person will notice almost instantly the effects of eating the calming foods and will experience a mental upsurge after eating energizing food.

Food allergies—special sensitivities to certain foods or food groups—are an altogether different matter. When you have an allergic reaction, your immune system *over*reacts to something in the food that your body perceives as a threat, and your defenses are mobilized out of all proportion to the "danger." (It's something like calling in the marines to do a traffic cop's job.) It is the overmobilization itself that constitutes the allergic reaction.

Food allergies aren't uncommon. But those that manifest themselves in mood swings and behavioral changes without accompanying physical symptoms, such as a stomachache, itchiness, a rash, or runny nose, are very rare. Recently both the American Medical Association and the Food and Drug Administration have issued statements to that effect. In other words, the experts who claim that people frequently feel hyper, anxious, or depressed as a result of an undiagnosed food allergy are usually wrong. And much of the advice in the books they have written is inaccurate and misleading.

If you suspect that you have a special sensitivity to a particular food, please see an allergist. But do keep in mind that if changes in the way you feel or behave after a meal are not accompanied by physical symptoms, those changes are probably a function of the food/mind/mood connection and *not* due to an allergy.

Once you learn the simple food strategies outlined in this book, you will be able to eat to direct the way you *want* to feel and perform.

Food/Mind/Mood Strategies and Blood Sugar

Just as mood and behavior changes that occur after eating are rarely the result of a food allergy, they also usually are unrelated to normal variations in blood sugar levels.

Many people believe they feel more energetic after eating a chocolate bar because the candy has raised their blood sugar level. However—and you had better sit down for this one—*all* the food/mind/mood research indicates that candy and other sugary foods are *calming*. In the next chapter, I will explain why people view candy as an energy food and how we now know that it actually tends to promote feelings of calmness and composure.

The important point for now is that in hundreds of laboratory studies in which our subjects' blood sugar levels were measured before eating, and at intervals afterward, we found very little connection in normal people between food, mood, and blood sugar levels. In test after test, we discovered that normal men and women feel less tense and anxious after eating the calming foods, regardless of whether their blood sugar goes up, down, or stays the same. We get the same results from the energizing foods.

Normal people feel more alert, vigorous, and motivated

after eating energizing foods, irrespective of changes in their blood sugar.

The exceptions are people who have been diagnosed as having hypoglycemia, a condition in which blood sugar levels are abnormally low. If you know you are hypoglycemic, you should check with your doctor and get an okay from him or her before following the food recommendations in this book.

Otherwise, understand that the ups and downs, the mental energy or lack of it, the grumpiness or easing of anxiety that you feel when you eat certain foods or avoid others are only indirectly related to variations in your blood sugar. Rather, they are the result of changes in your brain chemistry.

Remember, some foods influence the brain to manufacture substances that calm. Other foods increase the production in the brain of substances that stimulate and energize. For the vast majority of people, changes in brain chemistry are far more important in their food/mind/mood response than changes in blood sugar.

You *can* manage your moods, boost your mental capabilities, and maximize your performance easily and almost instantly by eating foods that have the desired effect on the chemistry of your brain!

2. Food/Mind/Mood Strategies— They're Safe

When I first explain the relation between food, mood, and brain chemicals to my patients, they often begin to look uneasy or doubtful. We tend to forget that our bodies are *made* of chemicals, instead thinking of chemicals as dangerous man-made substances that can poison us and pollute the environment. The brain, on the other hand, is rightly perceived by most people as the most complex, fragile, and essential of organs. So when I use those two words together— *chemicals* and *brain*—I can sometimes almost hear the alarm bells going off in people's heads.

I want to reassure you, as I have reassured them, that there is absolutely zero risk in the food/mind/mood strategies I've developed. The mood-modifying chemicals involved, including dopamine, norepinephrine, and serotonin (more about them in the next chapter) are already present in your brain, and their production is in a constant state of flux.

In following my recommendations, you will not be introducing any new or foreign substances into your body. Nor will you be inducing any unusual changes in the chemical processes that normally take place in your brain. You *will* be harnessing those processes, using them to achieve more of what you want at work and in your personal life.

As for the foods you will be using when you follow these food/mind/mood guidelines, they will be the ordinary, everyday foods you have always eaten and enjoyed. The only difference is that you may be eating some of them at times or in sequences that are new to you.

You will be doing nothing more risky or unnatural than, say, eating a bran muffin or some cottage cheese—but at the right time and in the right sequence.

And if you don't like bran muffins or cottage cheese? No problem. As you'll soon discover, there are dozens and dozens of other mood- and mind-enhancing foods with similar properties that you *will* like.

Food/Mind/Mood Strategies— They're Fast-Acting

These food/mind/mood strategies will work when you want them to, whenever you want them to. And by that I mean there's no "preconditioning" period of days or weeks during which your body must become accustomed to a new way of eating before it will respond. On the contrary, if you are like most people, your brain chemistry will react quickly and automatically to the appropriate foods the first and every time you use them to alter your moods, power your mind, and improve your performance.

How quickly? The changes in the way you feel and act after eating one of the mood-modifying foods often occur within half an hour, although if you are like me, you may notice the effects even sooner!

For example, I frequently begin to feel distracted and irritable late in the afternoon, and often by four-thirty or so I'm tempted to procrastinate—to clear off my desk and put off until tomorrow what really should be done today. But within fifteen minutes after eating my favorite calming, focusing food (Cheerios—no milk!), I'm back on track and eager to push on with my work until dinner at seven or seven-thirty.

Some people respond even more quickly—in a fast five minutes, in fact.

But whatever your normal food/mind/mood response interval might be, I've developed a special speed-up technique that you can use when you want or need to experience the quickest possible results. This technique shaves crucial minutes off the time it usually takes to get the appropriate food into your system and produce the essential changes in your brain chemistry. I will be describing it in detail in chapter 13.

Food/Mind/Mood Strategies— They're Proven

Scientific investigation of the relationship of food intake to mood, mental capabilities, and behavior has been carried out at several research institutions, first with laboratory animals and later with the help of many volunteer test subjects— healthy men and women of all ages and from practically every conceivable walk of life.

The usual test goes something like this: A group of volunteers comes to the lab and fills out questionnaires specially designed to pinpoint their mood states. Then each volunteer is given a meal. Some of them get meals consisting primarily of the calming foods; others get the mentally energizing foods. Then once an hour for three hours after eating, additional mood-testing questionnaires are filled out. (Volunteers, of course, are aware that we are studying their response to foods, but they do not know what their responses should be.)

Those who eat the calming foods consistently report feeling more relaxed, more focused, less stressed, less distracted after their meal. Behavioral tests rating performance on a number of tasks are also administered during the session. These tests confirm the volunteers' subjective assessments of their moods.

Those who eat the energizing foods report feeling more alert and motivated after their meal, and *their* performance tests show speedier responses and increased accuracy.

Naturally, there are individual variations in the food/mind/mood response. In some people, mood and performance ratings change dramatically after eating, while in others the differences are more subtle. And when we test the same volunteers on different occasions under somewhat different circumstances, we often find that their food/mind/mood response varies in intensity from one session to the next.

Nevertheless, these tests confirm a definite, measurable relationship between what one eats and how one feels and performs.

In chapter 4 you will find a questionnaire similar to those psychologists have developed for our volunteers at M.I.T. Use it to test your own food/mind/mood response. I think you will be fascinated by the results and what they reveal about you and your reactions to the food you eat.

The eating suggestions and guidelines in this book are, as noted, based on the results of experiments administered by scientific researchers at M.I.T. and elsewhere. They've worked for hundreds of people who have tried them. They'll work for you, too!

3. Food, Mood, and the Brain

"Just tell me what I'm supposed to eat, and I'll eat it."
As a nutritional counselor, I hear these words often. They reflect the results-oriented attitude of so many of the people who come to me for help with food-related problems.

Many of these men and women seek me out at my office in Cambridge, Massachusetts, because they've heard about our research on food, mind, mood, and performance, and they're eager to get started on a power eating program of their own. Others are referred by psychiatrists and physicians who suspect that there may be a nutritional component to their patients' feelings of stress, anxiety, or mental lethargy.

But no matter how they find their way to our office, when clients say, "Just tell me what to eat and I'll eat it," I know what it means: They're not interested in scientific explanations about food and the way it affects brain chemistry, as long as the eating guidelines work.

Obviously, my main interest also is in giving advice that works. But in my view, nutritional counseling is more than just prescribing. It should involve the hows and whys as well as the dos and don'ts, because I am convinced that when clients understand *why* I tell them to eat in a particular way, they achieve much better results.

It's the same with you. If you know *how* what you eat influences your moods, your mind, and your performance—if you know *why* I suggest eating certain foods in certain circumstances and other foods at other times—you will get the best possible results from the easy-to-follow strategies in the chapters to come. That's why I want you to read this chapter carefully, for it reveals how various foods affect your brain chemistry. I promise to simplify and make the science as brief and painless as possible. (For those of you with a science background or who want to learn more about the chemical basis of the food/mind/mood response, I've included a bibliography at the back of the book.)

Ready? Here goes.

The Mood-Modifying Chemicals— Dopamine, Norepinephrine, and Serotonin

In the brain, messages—small chunks of information—are passed from cell to cell by means of electrical impulses and chemicals. The chemicals are called *neurotransmitters*. More than a decade ago, it was discovered that three of the chemical neurotransmitters are manufactured by the brain from constituents of the food we eat. These three chemical neurotransmitters are dopamine, norepinephrine, and serotonin.

Because of their molecular structure, the first two are classified as catecholamines. (Adrenaline is another example of a catecholamine.) Serotonin, the third neurotransmitter that the brain synthesizes from food, is classified as an indoleamine, based on its molecular structure.

Dopamine and norepinephrine are the alertness chemicals. Research done with laboratory animals and with human volunteers indicates that when the brain is producing dopamine and norepinephrine, distinct changes in mood and behavior take place. In people these changes include a tendency to think more quickly, react more rapidly to stimuli, and feel more attentive, motivated, and mentally energetic. Problems, even big ones, often seem more manageable because of heightened "brain power." Practically everyone has had that marvelous feeling of being on a mental roll, when everything just sort of clicks into place in your mind. Well, when you experience that feeling, it's the dopamine and norepinephrine at work in your brain.

Serotonin is the calming chemical. Lab studies show the effects of serotonin to be quite different from those of dopamine and norepinephrine. When the brain is actively using serotonin, feelings of stress and tension are eased and the ability to concentrate is enhanced. When your thoughts seem to spin off in all directions at once, an increase of serotonin in the brain will act as a sort of brake, allowing you to filter out distractions and focus more sharply on the job at hand. Serotonin also slows reaction time somewhat and, depending on the time of day, may make you feel sluggish or sleepy.

Introducing the Amino Acids, Prime Ingredients of the Mood-Modifying Chemicals

Your brain synthesizes dopamine, norepinephrine, and serotonin from amino acids. If you have read books and magazine articles about nutrition—or remember Biology I in college—you know that amino acids are the nitrogen-containing chemicals from which proteins are "built." Proteins, in turn, are often referred to as "the building blocks of life," since every cell is made at least in part of protein. You also know that protein is an essential nutrient, supplied by foods of animal origin, legumes (peas, beans), grains, seeds, and nuts.

There are many different types of proteins, each made up of

amino acids in various combinations. In this brief discussion of the food/mind/mood response, we are concerned with only two amino acids:

- *Tyrosine, the principal ingredient in the neurotransmitters dopamine and norepinephrine.* When tyrosine from the food you eat enters your brain, and your brain is rapidly using up its present supply of dopamine and norepinephrine, production of the alertness chemicals is stimulated.
- *Tryptophan, the amino acid from which the neurotransmitter serotonin is made.* Whenever tryptophan is delivered to your brain, more serotonin, the calming chemical, is manufactured.

Since the protein foods you eat contain both tyrosine and tryptophan, it stands to reason that the more protein you take in, the more of both of these important amino acids will be available to your brain. But nature has a logic of her own.

Tyrosine, Protein, and the Alertness Effect

It's certainly true that whenever you eat protein, more tyrosine will reach your brain. It doesn't matter what kind of protein you eat or whether you eat it alone (as in an unadorned slice of white meat chicken, for example) or in combination with a carbohydrate food such as bread (as in a chicken sandwich). Getting protein into your system, either all by itself or with an accompanying carbohydrate, *always* makes more tyrosine available to your brain.

When there is ample tyrosine for your brain to draw upon— and if dopamine and norepinephrine are rapidly being used up—your brain will use the tyrosine to make more of the two alertness chemicals.

In general, then, eating protein foods increases alertness and has an energizing effect on your mind.

Tryptophan, Carbohydrates, and the Calming Effect

Simply eating protein will get more tyrosine into your brain, but this is not the case with tryptophan. Even though it is an amino acid, like tyrosine, and present in protein foods, just eating more protein will *not* increase the supply of tryptophan to your brain.

How come? Tyrosine, tryptophan, and four—count 'em, four—other amino acids present in protein foods all enter the brain via a common pathway, a special structure on the membrane surrounding the brain. But since space on the pathway is limited, all six amino acids cannot just zip into the brain at once.

To understand the phenomenon, it helps to compare the pathway by which these amino acids enter the brain to the ramps leading onto a major highway. Imagine that the amino acids are cars that must maneuver into position on a ramp before they can gain access to the highway. After eating protein, your body is flooded with amino acids, all competing for space on the ramp leading to the highway to the brain. Of the six amino acids, tryptophan is least plentiful, thus the ramps quickly fill up with the other five, and little or no tryptophan manages to get through to the brain.

How do we know this? In measuring the concentration of various amino acids in the brains of laboratory animals after they've been fed protein, researchers find no net increase in the amount of tryptophan. In fact, after a few days of being fed nothing but protein, lab animals actually show a net *loss* of tryptophan from their brains. An all-protein diet, in other words, actually depletes the supply of tryptophan in the animals' brains. It is the same with human beings.

But if eating protein won't increase the availability of the amino acid tryptophan to the brain, then what will?

The answer, surprisingly enough, is to eat *carbohydrates*—alone, without protein.

Carbohydrate, eaten either as a sweet food like jam or a starchy food such as bread or pasta, triggers the release of insulin from the pancreas. Insulin, of course, helps regulate blood sugar levels. However, another important but lesser-known function is to keep the amino acids from the food we eat moving through the bloodstream to rendezvous with cells throughout the body.

As the various amino acids leave the bloodstream to join up with bone, muscle, lung, and other organ cells, tryptophan—which tends to be "anchored" to albumin in the blood—keeps

The Food/Mind/Mood Response in a Nutshell

Dopamine, norepinephrine, serotonin, and the amino acids tyrosine and tryptophan all have important roles in producing the food/mind/mood response. But the key points for you to keep in mind from now on, the principles that underlie all the mood-managing and power eating strategies to come, are these:

• If you eat protein either alone or with a carbohydrate and your brain is rapidly using up its supply of dopamine and norepinephrine, it will use tyrosine supplied by the protein to manufacture more of these two neurotransmitters. When that happens, you'll find yourself responding more quickly and with greater accuracy to mental challenges. You will be more alert, more motivated, more mentally energetic and "up."

• If you eat carbohydrate alone, without protein, more tryptophan will be made available to your brain, which will use it to make more serotonin. As a result, you will feel less stressed, less anxious, more focused and relaxed.

on circulating. Soon there is more tryptophan in relation to other amino acids in the blood, and with less competition from the other amino acids, tryptophan easily finds a place on that ramp that leads to the highway to the brain.

To recap, when carbohydrates are eaten "straight," without protein, insulin is released into the bloodstream, which is then quickly emptied of other amino acids. The way is then opened for tryptophan to make its move up the ramp and on into the brain, where it will be used to manufacture serotonin, the calming chemical.

Eating carbohydrates alone, without protein, has a calming, focusing effect.

"Natural" Amino Acids Versus Those That Come in a Bottle

If you've ever browsed the shelves of a health food store, you may have noticed that both tyrosine and tryptophan are available in pill form. You might even, after reading the preceding paragraphs, be tempted to run out and buy some. Please don't. To begin with, the FDA has not given permission for these two amino acids to be sold or prescribed as a drug. And if you take them out of a bottle, not as they come in food, you will be taking them like a drug.

To take either or both of the amino acids in their most concentrated form, from a bottle, is to put yourself at risk for some potentially harmful side effects. Excessive amounts of concentrated tyrosine, for example, can cause undesirable changes in blood pressure. Too much concentrated tryptophan can result in extreme drowsiness or dizziness, making it difficult to carry out the simplest everyday tasks and posing very real hazards when driving a car or operating other machinery.

Further, large doses of either of these amino acids in concentrated form can inhibit entry into the brain of the other one—they cancel each other out. Indeed, they can block access to the brain of any or all of the five essential amino acids necessary for good health.

Your body has its own efficient system for regulating the production and activity of these two amino acids. It takes as much of each as it can use when you eat, and any excess is safely stored or eliminated. It is impossible to overdose on the amino acids in food. Nature designed the system. The system works, and by following the food guidelines in later chapters, you can help it work even better!

Choosing Foods for Best Results

As you might imagine, not all protein or carbohydrate foods will give you the same sure, quick mood-modifying and performance-boosting results. Some are better than others. The best tend to be those that can be eaten in their purest form.

Proteins

As you know, all proteins are made up of amino acids. But nature rarely packages the foods that contain large amounts of amino acids (meat, fish, dairy products, and protein-rich vegetables such as peas, peanuts, lentils, soybeans, etc.) in biochemically pure form.

For example, the white of an egg is perhaps the purest of all the protein foods in that it is composed entirely of amino acids and contains no fat and no carbohydrates. But the *yolk* of an egg is mainly fat. Thus, though whole eggs are classified as "protein foods," they are certainly not pure protein.

Does this mean you must eat bowls of egg whites in order to coax your brain to make more of the alertness chemicals?

No . . . fortunately. But it is important to choose protein foods that contain only small amounts of fats and/or carbohydrates when you want to shift quickly into a more alert, energetic, and motivated state of mind.

THE "A" LIST. Best bets because they contain very little fat and almost no carbohydrates are the following foods, listed here in no particular order:

Shellfish
Fish
Chicken (without the skin, which has a high fat content)
Veal
Very lean beef trimmed of all visible fat

THE "B" LIST. Almost as good are low-fat dairy products and vegetable protein sources, which are also very low in fat. Although vegetable protein sources are often also high in carbohydrates, they contain enough of the amino acid tyrosine to spur production of the alertness chemicals. All of those listed below are equally useful:

Low-fat cottage cheese
Skimmed or low-fat milk
Low-fat yogurt
Dried peas and beans
Lentils
Tofu and other soybean-based foods

THE "C" LIST. The following foods are high in protein but also relatively high in fat. And since the fat tends to slow their rate of absorption into the system, they should not be counted on to produce quick results. During the long, drawn out digestive process that follows a high-fat meal, relatively more blood is diverted *to* the stomach and intestines and *away* from the brain. Mental processes are slowed, the mind is dulled, and the result is sloppy thinking . . . or no thinking at all, as lethargy and even drowsiness set in.

So, although fat doesn't affect the brain in quite the same way as proteins and carbohydrates, which induce chemical changes, it does influence mind, mood, and performance—and always in negative ways.

Fat also adds to the calorie content of foods, a factor to keep in mind if you are concerned about weight. Don't count on any of the high-fat-content protein foods below to trigger an increase in mental energy. Most will *do the opposite!*

Beef (unless well trimmed of fat; keep in mind that "prime" beef tends to be higher in fat content than lesser grades)
Lamb
Pork and pork products (sausage, bacon, etc.)
Lunch meats (cold cuts), unless they are clearly labeled "low-fat"
Organ meats (liver, tongue, etc.)
Hard cheeses
Whole milk
Regular yogurt (as opposed to low-fat varieties)

Carbohydrates

Quick nutrition lesson: The foods loosely categorized as carbohydrates are of two basic types: *sugars,* which nutritionists often refer to as *simple carbohydrates,* and *starches,* which technically are known as *complex carbohydrates.* The adjectives *simple* and *complex* describe the molecular structures of these organic compounds. Sugars, in other words, are made up of less complex molecules than starches.

The most effective carbohydrate for getting your brain to make more serotonin is one you probably won't encounter in pure form except when you are undergoing certain medical tests or need to be fed intravenously: glucose.

Glucose is a sugar, one of several different types of sugar (some others are sucrose, fructose, and lactose). According to scientists, it is the *only* sugar capable of causing an immediate increase in the amount of insulin released by the pancreas. (Increased insulin, remember, is crucial to the process by which tryptophan gains access to the brain and stimulates the production of serotonin.)

Consuming pure glucose is about as appealing as eating

plain egg whites. But again, lucky for us, most carbohydrates—simple and complex—have enough glucose in their makeup to activate the food-mood response.

SWEETS. Table sugar (sucrose) is chemically part glucose and part fructose; so are the corn sweeteners used to flavor many commercial goodies. And so is honey. Thus, almost any sweet-tasting food made with a relatively large amount of table sugar, corn sweetener, or honey contains glucose and will initiate the complicated process that ends with the brain making more serotonin. A list of these foods reads like a compendium of no-nos for dieters, but as you will soon see, it doesn't take much to produce the desired effect.

Candy
Cookies
Pie
Cake
Ice cream
Jams, jellies, and preserves
Syrup
Soft drinks

Fruit won't activate the food/mind/mood response. The sweet taste of fruits and fruit juices is due to their high fructose content. (Fructose, as it happens, is the sweetest of all the sugars—gram for gram *much* sweeter than sucrose.) But although fructose is eventually converted into glucose by the body, the process is so slow and so gradual that fruit is practically useless for promoting serotonin production. Fruit is good for you, no doubt about it. But don't reach for an apple or an orange when you want to feel more focused or less stressed. It won't work.

STARCHES. Products made of wheat, corn, and other types of flour, as well as the vegetables commonly referred to as "starchy" (such as potatoes), are chemically composed of long chains of glucose molecules. Upon entering the blood from the intestinal tract, where digestion occurs, the glucose in these foods triggers the release of insulin, allowing tryptophan to reach the brain and thereby stimulating the production of serotonin. Eating any of the following grains and starches will help you achieve a calmer, more focused state of mind:

Bread
Crackers, muffins, rolls, bagels
Pasta
Potatoes
Rice
Corn (including tortillas)
Barley
Kasha
Oatmeal and other cereals. (However, if you add milk to oatmeal or any other cereal, you are introducing a protein, which will inhibit the manufacture of serotonin.)

Leafy greens and bright-colored vegetables are food-mood "neutral." Lettuce, spinach, broccoli, carrots, beets, and the other vitamin-rich, low-calorie vegetables are part of a well-balanced diet, and I hope you will eat them as often as possible. However, they do not supply complex carbohydrates in amounts large enough to spur your brain to make more serotonin. In this regard, half a baked potato is worth a whole plateful of spinach.

The Fat Factor

In the following chapters I will explain the techniques that will enable you to manage your mind and your moods and perform up to your best potential in various situations and circumstances. I will suggest that you eat meals and snacks that are high in protein in order to master some kinds of challenges. Meeting other demands will require an emphasis on carbohydrates.

Nowhere in this book will I urge you to eat high-fat foods.

In fact, time and again I will remind you to avoid butter, mayonnaise, fried foods, fatty meats, hard cheeses, creamed soups, and rich gravies and sauces.

There are a number of good reasons to keep fat intake as low as possible. Fat has been linked to the development of killer diseases such as heart disease, stroke, and certain types of cancer. And then, of course, fat is higher in calories than other food elements—gram for gram more than twice as high as protein and carbohydrate! Thus, high-fat foods are always high-calorie foods and to be avoided by all but the extremely underweight.

More important from the food/mind/mood point of view, fat takes longer to digest than other foods, and that affects your mood and mind negatively, as we've already noted.

How Much Protein, How Much Carbohydrate Is Enough?

In working with laboratory animals, it is easy to determine the amount of protein it takes to increase production of dopamine and norepinephrine in their brains. We simply feed the animals varying amounts of protein food and then measure the resulting changes in their brain chemistry. We do the same to find out how much carbohydrate is necessary to increase serotonin levels.

For obvious reasons, we can't go into the brains of our human volunteers to get accurate data on chemical changes. But we can, and do, measure changes in the amino acid content of their blood after they have eaten specific amounts of protein or carbohydrate, and then calculate how much of the amino acids will ultimately reach their brains. These calculations, along with performance tests administered before and after volunteers have consumed different "dosages" of protein or carbohydrate, allow us to make a good estimate of the amounts necessary to bring about the food-mood response.

Here's what we have learned.

For most people, three to four ounces of a protein food delivers enough tyrosine to the brain to stimulate production of dopamine and norepinephrine, the alertness chemicals that keep you mentally up, thinking quickly and accurately, with the brain power to tackle any challenges that come your way.

As little as one or one and a half ounces of a carbohydrate food—a sweet or starch—will allow enough tryptophan to enter your brain to increase the manufacture of serotonin, the calming chemical that enhances powers of concentration and eases feelings of anxiety and frustration. The only individuals who may need *more* carbohydrates in order to trigger serotonin production are those who are 20 percent or more over their ideal weight and women in the days just prior to menstruation. For these two groups, two or two and a half ounces of carbohydrate food may be required. But unless you belong in one of these categories, an ounce of a sweet or starchy food is all you need to feel more focused and more relaxed and less easily distracted and less fidgety or stressed, regardless of whether you are tall or short, young or old, male or female.

If a little is good, will more protein or carbohydrate produce even better results? It is a question almost everyone asks sooner or later, and the answer is no.

The mood mechanisms of your brain are so finely tuned that even a small chemical change will make a noticeable difference in the way you feel, think, and perform. But, with a few exceptions that I will explain later, the effects of food on mind and mood appear to be self-limiting. Doubling your protein intake won't make you feel twice as alert; doubling your carbohydrate intake won't make you concentrate twice as well. Only your calorie count for the day will be affected.

But Does It Always Work?

Can you count on the food/mind/mood response every single time?

The answer, basically, is yes, although with a minor qualification or two. (My colleagues and I all have experienced these phenomena ourselves.)

Eating protein either alone or with some carbohydrate will result in an increase of the alertness chemicals dopamine and norepinephrine *if* your brain is using up its current supply and needs to replace them. However, when your brain has ample amounts of the alertness chemicals to draw upon, eating protein won't stimulate it to produce more.

But, keep in mind that each time you eat protein, you are increasing the amount of tyrosine and other amino acids in your body, in effect preventing tryptophan from gaining access to your brain (because of increased competition for a place in the pathway to the brain). When the supply of tryptophan is blocked, your brain can't manufacture the calming chemical serotonin. This means that you will continue to be "up." So the effects of eating protein may be direct, as when it causes an increase in the alertness chemicals, or indirect, as when it inhibits the manufacture of serotonin.

Eating carbohydrate alone will always allow more tryptophan to reach your brain and will always result in increased production of serotonin.

That's the story, but it's not quite the whole story. Most of my patients and the volunteers involved in food-mood testing at M.I.T. and elsewhere find that they are more or less sensitive to what they eat at certain predictable times of the day. Chances are that it will be the same for you.

That's why learning how to set your own personal food-mood "clock"—which I will explain in the next section—is so important to the success of the food strategies and guidelines throughout this book.

But before we go on to the techniques of power eating in the morning, afternoon, and evening, why not test the food-mood response for yourself?

4. Testing Your Food/Mind/Mood Response

If you are of a skeptical turn of mind, as I and most scientists tend to be, you won't be 100 percent convinced that foods can have a dramatic effect on mood, mind, and performance until you experience some of these effects yourself. The food/mind/mood tests in this chapter will give you the opportunity to do just that.

These tests, with you as guinea pig, are similar to those that dozens of other scientific investigators and I have given to volunteers at M.I.T., at the National Institutes of Health, and at other research centers where studies on food and its influences on the brain are carried out. But there are two important differences.

First, of course, is the fact that our lab tests were carefully controlled experiments. Volunteers came to the test centers, answered questions about their state of mind on arrival, ate the food we gave them, and then answered the same questions again every hour or so for three hours after their meal. They were *never* briefed on how others before them responded or on how they themselves might be expected to respond. (But you already know something of what to expect if you just finished reading the preceding chapter.)

Most people are more or less susceptible to the power of suggestion, and you probably are no exception. If a student, for example, is told often enough that economics is a boring, dry subject, it increases the likelihood that he or she will find economics intolerably dull when the time comes to study it. In the same way, if you fully expect to feel mentally pepped up and invigorated after eating protein and more relaxed and focused after eating carbohydrate, your anticipation of these changes may indeed influence your perceptions.

Does all this invalidate the results of experiments you are about to make? If the aim were to confirm an untested hypothesis, I would have to answer that question with a yes.

But, remember, we already have reams of scientific data on the food/mind/mood response. The object of your own experiments is not to gather more confirming data, it is to demonstrate your sensitivity to protein and carbohydrate and allow you to feel their effects firsthand.

Frankly, I can't promise that some of what you feel after eating the test meals and snacks won't be the result of your own suggestibility. But I *can* guarantee that *most* of what you feel will be due to changes in your brain chemistry, triggered by the amino acids tyrosine and tryptophan.

The second way in which the tests on the next few pages differ from our lab experiments is that, in working with volunteers, we never rely solely on how they *say* they feel after eating a protein- or carbohydrate-based meal. Their subjective impressions are always backed up by objective performance tests.

For example, there are reaction-time tests. If you were a volunteer at M.I.T., you probably would be asked to take one of these. You would be fitted with earphones and told to keep your finger pressed down on a button, lifting it as quickly as possible each time you heard a tone through the earphones. In these tests, protein-eating volunteers tend to react quickly and accurately to the occasional random tones. Carbohydrate eaters, on the other hand, usually exhibit markedly slower reaction time and make more errors, either failing to lift their fingers on cue or lifting them *before* they hear a tone.

Another type of test, called a vigilance test, measures the ability to stay alert over long periods of time. Earphones are used for this one, too. But in vigilance testing, you hear a series of one-second tones, interspersed at random with a few slightly shorter tones, lasting, say, three-quarters of a second. Subjects are told to press a button only when they hear the shorter tone. Since this test lasts a full sixty minutes, it can be a real endurance contest. Once again, the protein eaters tend to do better than the more relaxed carbohydrate eaters. In fact, often when I monitor vigilance testing sessions, I am amused to see the carbohydrate eaters, eyelids drooping, slump lower and lower in their chairs as the minutes tick by. Once we actually had to wake a volunteer who had dozed off for a blissful late-afternoon snooze.

In still another test done with earphones, a string of words broken up into their component sounds and syllables is spoken right into a subject's ear. For instance, the word *picturesque* might come through as *p - ictu - r - esk*. As the subject hears the sounds, he or she must repeat them to the tester, who is sitting nearby. After several minutes of this—and without any warning—the subject will suddenly hear a second voice in his or her left ear, reciting nonsense syllables totally different from those spoken into the right ear. This is called a "distraction message," and the object is to block it out while continuing to repeat the sounds and syllables directed to the right ear. Results of this test are fascinating. Although carbohydrate-eating volunteers consistently make more errors *before* the second voice comes through, they are better able to ignore the distraction message than the protein eaters. And this confirms what many people have told us verbally and in questionnaires about their mental state after eating carbohydrate. Although they felt somewhat less sharp, they believed their ability to concentrate had improved!

It would be ideal if I could somehow include with the food/mind/mood demonstration questionnaires a few sample performance tests such as the one we give our volunteers at the M.I.T. testing center. That way, you could double-check your responses after eating protein or carbohydrate, verifying your subjective feelings with your scores on objective tests that require quick thinking and reacting, alertness, concentration, etc. But obviously it is impossible to duplicate these tests without special equipment and a trained tester to measure the results.

In fact, objective testing really isn't necessary when your goal is to manage your mind and your moods with food.

Once you learn the techniques of power eating and the strategies that will enable you to function at peak in any situation—whether it requires split-second responses and a high degree of mental accuracy or calls for a calmer, more focused approach—you will discover that the food strategies in this book are self-verifying. Just use them, and you'll see!

Self-Testing Dos and Don'ts

These tests are designed to help you determine your sensitivity to eating protein and carbohydrate at different times of the day. You won't be able to run through all of them in one day, since I want you to try out *two* kinds of meals—high-protein and high-carbohydrate—for breakfast, lunch, and dinner. I also want you to experience changes in the way you think and feel after eating protein and carbohydrates at times when you are most likely to snack.

There are a few rules you must follow to make the test results as valid as possible:

1. Eat the test meals and snacks on ordinary days when you do not anticipate doing anything unusual, either professionally or socially, and when your schedule is apt to be routine. (If workdays are often filled with unexpected demands, it may be a good idea to plan test meals and snacks for weekends—or vice versa.)

2. Schedule the two test breakfasts for the same time slot on each test morning; do the same for the lunches, dinners, and snacks. The reason: Time of day can affect the way you respond to food. For example, if you eat a protein test lunch at, say, noon on Monday and the carbohydrate test lunch at two-thirty on Wednesday, the mood and mental performance differences you notice after meals may be distorted by time variations.

3. Keep caffeine intake consistent with what is normal for you. If you are accustomed to drinking several cups of coffee or tea daily, do not drink more or less when you take a food/mind/mood test. However, do *not* drink a caffeinated beverage less than two hours before a test meal or snack, and do not drink any with your meal or snack. Wait until one and a half hours after. As you will see when you read the chapter on caffeine, it can have a powerful effect on how you think and feel and can skew test meal results.

4. Do not drink alcoholic beverages on test days.

5. Avoid all beverages and foods flavored with NutraSweet on test days, because we do not know its effect on mood, mind, or behavior.

6. Eat only the foods suggested for each test meal or snack.

7. Since it is extremely important to eat a test meal when your stomach is empty, wait at least four hours after breakfast before you eat a test lunch, and forego a midmorning snack on that day. For the same reason, wait at least four hours after lunch before you eat a test dinner, and do not eat a midafternoon snack between the two meals.

8. For valid results, the meal preceding a test snack or meal *must be low in fat*.

How to Determine Your Own Food/Mind/Mood Response

Now, here's how to take the test and measure your sensitivity to proteins and carbohydrates at various times of day:

• No more than fifteen minutes before each test meal or snack, rate your mood or state of mind *at that moment*. Do it by placing a 0, 1, or 2 next to each of the descriptive words in the "before meal" column of the questionnaire. Use 0 for adjectives that do not apply, 1 for those that apply only slightly, and 2 when the feeling is intense.

Be as accurate and honest as possible, but work quickly. In other words, don't stop to ruminate over each word in the column. Your first, off-the-top-of-the-head response probably will be a more accurate reflection of your true state of mind than an answer arrived at after moments of soul-searching.

• An hour after your demonstration meal or snack, rate your state of mind again by placing a 0, 1, or 2 next to each of the adjectives in the "after meal" column of the questionnaire.

To make it easier to write in your responses to the test menus that follow, copy them into an 8½″ × 11″ notebook, either by hand or by photocopying these pages and stapling the copies into your notebook. You also will find this convenient to carry with you when you eat your test meals away from home.

You may wish to confirm your results by repeating these tests. If you do, try to repeat them in circumstances as much the same as possible. Weigh your responses as objectively as you can, rating your state of mind without reflecting on your previous "test results." Wait to compare until after you've completed the repeat test.

Breakfast Test I—Protein

Start the day with:
8-ounce container plain low-fat yogurt *or*
5 ounces low-fat cottage cheese *or*
2 soft-boiled, poached, scrambled, or fried eggs. (Use a nonstick pan
   and no butter or margarine for scrambling or frying eggs, or try a
   no-cal, nonstick spray.)

4–6 ounces fruit juice *or*
1 piece fruit, such as an orange, apple, pear, etc.

Coffee or tea as usual, with milk if desired. (Use no sugar and no
   artificial sweeteners but saccharine.)

State of Mind	Before Meal	After Meal
Alert		
Vigorous		
Energetic		
Motivated		
Quick		
Relaxed		
Calm		
Patient		
Focused		
Irritable		
Grouchy		
Agitated		
Tense		
Shaky		
Sluggish		
Apathetic		
Slow		
Sleepy		
Sad		
Blue		
Despairing		
Unable to cope		

Breakfast Test II—Carbohydrate

Soon after awakening, have:

1 muffin, bagel, or English muffin *or*

2 slices toast with 1 teaspoon jelly *or*

2 medium pancakes or waffles, with 1 tablespoon syrup or jelly (no butter) *or*

1–1½ cups hot or cold cereal without milk

Coffee or tea as usual, with sugar if desired, but with no more than 2 tablespoons milk. (Use no artificial sweeteners other than saccharine.)

State of Mind	Before Meal	After Meal
Alert		
Vigorous		
Energetic		
Motivated		
Quick		
Relaxed		
Calm		
Patient		
Focused		
Irritable		
Grouchy		
Agitated		
Tense		
Shaky		
Sluggish		
Apathetic		
Slow		
Sleepy		
Sad		
Blue		
Despairing		
Unable to cope		

Lunch Test I—Protein

At the time you usually break for lunch, have one of the following combinations:

3–4 ounces cold chicken, turkey, lean roast beef, or lean cold cuts
   and
2 cups raw vegetables (carrots, green peppers, tomatoes, etc.)

3-ounce can tuna (water-packed or well drained of oil) *and*
1½ cups green salad

2 hard-boiled eggs *and*
1½ cups lettuce and tomato salad

6–8 ounces cottage cheese or low-fat yogurt *with*
1 piece of fruit, sliced (banana, pear, peach, apple—or 1 cup berries)

State of Mind	Before Meal	After Meal
Alert		
Vigorous		
Energetic		
Motivated		
Quick		
Relaxed		
Calm		
Patient		
Focused		
Irritable		
Grouchy		
Agitated		
Tense		
Shaky		
Sluggish		
Apathetic		
Slow		
Sleepy		
Sad		
Blue		
Despairing		
Unable to cope		

Lunch Test II—Carbohydrate

At your normal lunch hour, choose one of the following:

2 cups pasta with plain tomato sauce (no meat or clam sauce)

1 large baked potato with no more than 1 tablespoon sour cream or butter *and*

1 roll or 2 slices of bread or 1 medium (6″) pita bread with 1 teaspoon jelly

2 cups Chinese fried rice *and*

12-ounce soft drink (regular, not diet)

1 peanut butter and jelly sandwich (with 1 tablespoon peanut butter and 2 tablespoons jelly) *and*

12-ounce soft drink (regular, not diet)

State of Mind	Before Meal	After Meal
Alert		
Vigorous		
Energetic		
Motivated		
Quick		
Relaxed		
Calm		
Patient		
Focused		
Irritable		
Grouchy		
Agitated		
Tense		
Shaky		
Sluggish		
Apathetic		
Slow		
Sleepy		
Sad		
Blue		
Despairing		
Unable to cope		

Dinner Test I—Protein

In the evening, have:
4–6 ounces broiled fish prepared with 1–2 teaspoons oil or butter *or*
4–6 ounces poultry or veal

1½ cups vegetables, such as green beans, asparagus, zucchini, yellow squash, broccoli, cauliflower, or tossed salad (with 1 teaspoon dressing)

1 piece fresh fruit for dessert

State of Mind	Before Meal	After Meal
Alert		
Vigorous		
Energetic		
Motivated		
Quick		
Relaxed		
Calm		
Patient		
Focused		
Irritable		
Grouchy		
Agitated		
Tense		
Shaky		
Sluggish		
Apathetic		
Slow		
Sleepy		
Sad		
Blue		
Despairing		
Unable to cope		

Dinner Test II—Carbohydrate

For your evening meal, have:

1–2 cups noodles or spaghetti with marinara sauce or plain tomato sauce *or*

2 cups rice mixed with cooked vegetables such as carrots, zucchini, green pepper, onion, green beans, cauliflower, broccoli, etc., *or*

1 large sweet or white potato, 1½ cups salad, and 2 slices garlic bread *or*

2–3 large slices pizza (without sausage or anchovies)

12-ounce can regular (not diet) soft drink with meal, if desired

1 piece fruit of any kind for dessert

State of Mind	Before Meal	After Meal
Alert		
Vigorous		
Energetic		
Motivated		
Quick		
Relaxed		
Calm		
Patient		
Focused		
Irritable		
Grouchy		
Agitated		
Tense		
Shaky		
Sluggish		
Apathetic		
Slow		
Sleepy		
Sad		
Blue		
Despairing		
Unable to cope		

Midmorning Snack Test I—Protein

At least two *hours after a low-fat breakfast, have:*
1 hard-boiled egg *or*
3–4 ounces cottage cheese or plain yogurt *or*
1 ounce low-fat cheese, such as skim-milk mozzarella or ricotta, *or*
2 ounces chicken or water-packed tuna

1 piece of fruit of any kind, if desired

State of Mind	Before Meal	After Meal
Alert		
Vigorous		
Energetic		
Motivated		
Quick		
Relaxed		
Calm		
Patient		
Focused		
Irritable		
Grouchy		
Agitated		
Tense		
Shaky		
Sluggish		
Apathetic		
Slow		
Sleepy		
Sad		
Blue		
Despairing		
Unable to cope		

Midmorning Snack Test II—Carbohydrate

At least two *hours after a low-fat breakfast, have:*
1 muffin, bagel, plain or sugar-coated doughnut, *or*
1 package peanut butter crackers (six to a package) *or*
1–2 ounces popcorn (no butter) *or*
5–6 graham crackers or vanilla wafers *or*
1–1½ cups dry cereal

State of Mind	Before Meal	After Meal
Alert		
Vigorous		
Energetic		
Motivated		
Quick		
Relaxed		
Calm		
Patient		
Focused		
Irritable		
Grouchy		
Agitated		
Tense		
Shaky		
Sluggish		
Apathetic		
Slow		
Sleepy		
Sad		
Blue		
Despairing		
Unable to cope		

Midafternoon Snack Test I—Protein

At least two hours after a small, low-fat lunch, have:
4–5 ounces cottage cheese or plain yogurt *or*
3 ounces sliced chicken or turkey (buy from deli or supermarket ahead of time) *or*
1–2 ounces low-fat cheese, such as skim-milk mozzarella or ricotta, *or*
3-ounce hamburger, no bun (if you are near a fast-food restaurant)

4–5 ounces fruit juice or 1 piece of fruit of any kind, if desired

State of Mind	Before Meal	After Meal
Alert		
Vigorous		
Energetic		
Motivated		
Quick		
Relaxed		
Calm		
Patient		
Focused		
Irritable		
Grouchy		
Agitated		
Tense		
Shaky		
Sluggish		
Apathetic		
Slow		
Sleepy		
Sad		
Blue		
Despairing		
Unable to cope		

Midafternoon Snack Test II—Carbohydrate

At least two *hours after a small, low-fat lunch, have:*
1–2 ounces popcorn (no butter) or pretzels *or*
1 medium bagel, corn or bran muffin, or 6″ pita bread with 1 teaspoon
    jelly, *or*
1 vending machine package of crackers or cookies *or*
1 large frozen yogurt cone *or*
1 ounce jelly beans or gumdrops *or*
1–1½ cups dry cereal

4–5 ounces fruit juice or 1 piece of fruit of any kind, if desired

State of Mind	Before Meal	After Meal
Alert		
Vigorous		
Energetic		
Motivated		
Quick		
Relaxed		
Calm		
Patient		
Focused		
Irritable		
Grouchy		
Agitated		
Tense		
Shaky		
Sluggish		
Apathetic		
Slow		
Sleepy		
Sad		
Blue		
Despairing		
Unable to cope		

Bedtime Snack Test I—Protein

At least two *hours after a low-fat dinner, have:*
3–4 ounces cooked lean meat (perhaps left over from dinner) *or*
2 poached, fried, or scrambled eggs (fry or scramble with butter or
    margarine in a nonstick pan, or use a nonstick spray) *or*
4–5 ounces low-fat cottage cheese or plain yogurt *or*
1–2 ounces of low-fat cheese, such as skim-milk mozzarella or ricotta

State of Mind	Before Meal	After Meal
Alert		
Vigorous		
Energetic		
Motivated		
Quick		
Relaxed		
Calm		
Patient		
Focused		
Irritable		
Grouchy		
Agitated		
Tense		
Shaky		
Sluggish		
Apathetic		
Slow		
Sleepy		
Sad		
Blue		
Despairing		
Unable to cope		

Bedtime Snack Test II—Carbohydrate

At least two *hours after a low-fat dinner, have:*
2 toaster-size waffles or pancakes with 1 tablespoon syrup or jam *or*
1 English muffin with 2 teaspoons jelly *or*
2 cups popcorn (no butter) sweetened with syrup or melted caramel,
    if desired, *or*
6 plain cookies or crackers *or*
8 toasted marshmallows *or*
1 cup herbal tea sweetened with 1 tablespoon sugar and 4 vanilla
    wafers

State of Mind	Before Meal	After Meal
Alert		
Vigorous		
Energetic		
Motivated		
Quick		
Relaxed		
Calm		
Patient		
Focused		
Irritable		
Grouchy		
Agitated		
Tense		
Shaky		
Sluggish		
Apathetic		
Slow		
Sleepy		
Sad		
Blue		
Despairing		
Unable to cope		

Interpreting Your
Food/Mind/Mood Test Scores

Obviously, if your score sheets show many changes of from 2 to 0 or 0 to 2 in your before- and after-meal state-of-mind ratings, food has a profound effect on the way you feel—and, by extension, on the way you perform, not only in routine everyday circumstances but also in those situations that demand the most of you professionally and personally. Your brain chemistry responds quickly and strongly to increases in the amounts of tyrosine and tryptophan it receives. For you, food can be an especially potent tool for managing your mind and your moods.

Just as obviously, if changes in your state of mind after eating are more subtle and less consistent—in other words, if your score sheets showed few leaps of from 0 to 2 or 2 to 0 but many smaller movements of a lesser degree (say, from 0 to 1 or 1 to 0), you are somewhat less sensitive to the food/mind/ mood response. For you, learning to take advantage of the mind- and mood-influencing capabilities of protein and carbohydrate can still make a difference between so-so performance and achieving your best potential. Just as important, mastering the techniques of eating to prevent food from working *against* you will give you an extra edge in the daily grind and boost your ability to function in top form when the going gets rough.

For Carbohydrate Cravers Only

Very few of our volunteers who were in good physical and mental health and complied fully with the instructions they were given during their test sessions experienced no state of mind changes after eating carbohydrates.

Some people exhibited a very specific response to, and need for, a carbohydrate snack. I call them "carbohydrate cravers." Perhaps you are one of them. You *are* if, before you ate your morning, afternoon, or evening test snacks, you rated your state of mind as irritable, grouchy, agitated, tense, or even shaky and then mellowed after a carbohydrate snack. On the day that you ate a protein test snack, your state of mind remained about the same, but on the day you ate a carbohydrate test snack, you rated yourself afterward as feeling more relaxed, calmer, patient, and more focused. People who are not carbohydrate cravers, on the other hand, tend to feel more apathetic, slowed-down, sluggish, or even sleepy after eating a carbohydrate-rich snack.

If your test results indicate that carbohydrates tend to *restore* your sense of well-being and enable you to settle down again, refocus on your work or whatever other activity you might have been engaged in, and in effect "go the extra mile," you are in the minority. Your food/mind/mood response is somewhat different from that of most other people. Your approach to managing your mind and your moods with food must, in a few instances, be different as well.

Here and there in the following chapters you will see the phrase *for carbohydrate cravers only*. If you are a carbohydrate craver, be sure to read carefully the special suggestions that follow. These suggestions are designed to help *you,* as a carbohydrate craver, gain even greater benefits from the mind- and mood-enhancing techniques in this book.

No One Is Immune!

But what if you noticed little or no change in your state of mind after eating protein or carbohydrate? Does it mean that you are immune to the food/mind/mood response? Is it pointless to experiment with the eating strategies that have helped so many of our clients become more productive, successful, and, in many cases, more content and fulfilled individuals?

Absolutely not! We *know* that food causes brain chemistry

changes that affect the way healthy men and women feel and perform. We also know that some people are more aware of their state of mind—more "in tune with their feelings," in other words—than others. In fact, I have treated dozens of clients who found it difficult to pinpoint variations in their moods but nevertheless began to feel and function better, and achieve more of what they wanted in their lives, when they followed the special food plans I worked out for them.

You may, like them, be less sensitive to the subtler mood changes yet responsive to power eating strategies all the same. But you never will know for sure unless you put those strategies into practice.

Whatever your scores reveal about the effect of protein and carbohydrate on your mental state, there is no better time than now to start managing your mind and your mood with food.

5. All-Day, Everyday Power Eating

Of course, you have heard the term *circadian rhythms*. It refers to the regular and predictable biological ups and downs in the body's mental and physical energy levels—cyclical peaks and valleys that repeat themselves every twenty-four hours or so, as regularly as dawn follows darkness and day slowly turns again into night.

To help you use food to power your brain, I'm going to tell you how to use what we know about food and its effect on brain chemistry so that you can enhance your biological cycles when they're on the upswing. I'm also going to tell you how to eat to keep mental energy levels high even when circadian rhythms are pushing them down. In this chapter you'll learn how to get the most out of every day. In the chapters that follow, I'll tell you how to adapt to the demands of days that require extra effort.

Your Internal "Clock"

Biological rhythms affect human beings, other animals, and even plants (circadian stimuli, for example, tell flowers to open their blooms wide with the coming of light each day). With regard to people, our internal circadian "clock" makes us feel relatively alert and mentally energetic during the first few hours after awakening. Later there is a natural slackening off in motivation and brain power, though the downhill slide in some people is steeper and more precipitous than in others. Finally, at the end of the day, usually within an hour or so before normal bedtime, there's a tendency to close up shop mentally.

If one were to draw a line illustrating the trend of mental energy over the sixteen or eighteen hours most of us are awake each day, it would be a downward slope, highest just after waking and gradually dropping down to sleep. Like this.

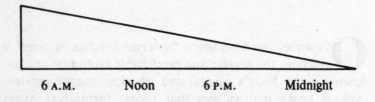

6 A.M.   Noon   6 P.M.   Midnight

It doesn't matter much whether you are a day person or a night person—a lark who bounces out of bed at five in the morning or earlier and then collapses back into the blankets at ten or eleven at night, or an owl who prefers to stay up for the "Late Late Show" and awaken at noon. Your mental energy and alertness will be highest in the first six or so hours after sleep. Then, little by little, there will be a tapering off to grogginess as the clock—the one on the wall as well as the internal mechanisms that regulate the many complex systems that make up your circadian rhythms—says it's time to go to bed.

Of course, there can be and are small blips within the larger pattern. We all have days when we stumble around half conscious until lunchtime, despite getting our usual amount of sleep. And on other days we feel mentally wide-awake and stimulated well past normal "closing time." But these are occasional variations on a much more basic theme and *may* (I emphasize the *may* because it is not always possible to know for sure) vary with the quantity, timing, and choice of foods consumed.

Circadian rhythms are powerful. They put your very cells on schedule, signaling glands when to increase or decrease production of certain hormones and influencing body temperature and energy expenditure. It's no wonder, then, that these natural rhythms also can have a profound effect on the way you feel and perform.

Thus, in planning a daily diet that will help you achieve your best potential on the job and in your personal life, it is important that the food you eat and the times at which you eat work with circadian rhythms whenever possible.

Equally important is using food to counteract biological rhythms so that you are able to maintain high performance levels even when the cycles that govern mental energy have begun to dip.

You might wonder how it is possible to counter your body's intrinsic rhythms successfully. Actually, it probably is easier than you think. In fact, it is likely that you already do it several times a day. For example, whenever you use an alarm clock instead of allowing yourself to sleep until your internal clock says that it is time to get up, you are interfering with your circadian rhythms. And every time you decide to engage in an evening activity that is mentally or physically stimulating—such as playing bridge, working late on a report, or swimming a few laps at the Y—you are asking your mind and body to ignore the biological tendency to decelerate at the end of the day.

Circadian rhythms are strong, but they can be overridden.

Food can influence your brain's production of the alertness chemicals, dopamine and norepinephrine, and the calming chemical, serotonin, giving you greater control over the cyclical ups and downs that affect the way you feel and perform.

Power eating helps you master biological ups and downs.

You can use the food/mind/mood response to accentuate the positive, maximizing mental energy and alertness when the biological cycles affecting your mind and body are peaking.

Conversely, you can use food to calm and relax you when your internal clock tells you to wind down but external pressures keep you tense and jumpy.

Most valuable of all, you can eat to neutralize temporarily the effects of circadian rhythms when they are signaling your body to slow down and unwind, and thus stretch out your productive hours, giving yourself an edge in meeting career and personal challenges.

In this chapter we are going to focus on power meals—breakfasts, lunches, and dinners—designed to increase mental effectiveness throughout the day. Since between-meal eating also plays an important role in mind and mood managing, I will also explain how to snack smarter.

The meal recommendations that follow were designed to help clients in my private practice power their brains and achieve higher performance levels on normal days, when demands at work and at home are not at crisis level (we'll get to that later). These guidelines have helped hundreds feel better and achieve more every day of their lives. I am convinced that you will find them equally helpful.

Breakfasts with Get-Up-and-Go

If you took the food/mind/mood tests in chapter 4, you may have found that breakfast—regardless of whether it was protein- or carbohydrate-based—had little effect on your state of mind. In scientific studies done with hundreds of volunteers, we discovered that most men and women who are not unduly stressed or physically fatigued do *not* experience drastic mind and mood changes after their morning meal.

Why do proteins and carbohydrates, which so quickly and effectively modify mind and mood later in the day, so often fail to do so in the morning?

The answer has to do with circadian rhythms. Remember, for most people most of the time, all systems are go early in the morning. Eating protein doesn't seem to increase alertness, motivation, and mental energy significantly, since mind and body are already revved up and in high gear. For the same reason, carbohydrates usually don't have a noticeably calming effect, since the wear, tear, and frustrations of the day haven't yet had a chance to get on your nerves.

Why You Must Eat a Good Breakfast

I insist that all my clients start every day with a good breakfast. I strongly urge you to do the same if you want to function in top form from the time you wake until the time you turn out the lights at night. Here's why:

• *Getting food into your system in the morning is "entraining."* (*Entraining* is a technical term referring to the support and enhancement of biological processes through synchronization.) Eating at a time when your body is switching from the lower energy expenditures, lower temperatures, and lower hormone production of the nighttime hours into its more active daytime mode helps make these transitions occur more smoothly and efficiently—and with better results for you. When supplied with the proper nutrients and energy just as circadian rhythms are about to peak, your body is a little like a runner with wind at his or her back—effortlessly able to go a little faster and a little farther than otherwise.

• *A good breakfast—or at least a nutritious snack before midday—will help prevent you from eating too much at lunch.* I've had a number of clients who never ate or drank anything but coffee until noon. Although many of them were able to get through the mornings without the discomfort and distraction of hunger pangs, they all approached lunch as though they hadn't encountered food for hours, which, of course, was exactly the case. The outsized lunches they then consumed resulted in calorie overload, which decreased their alertness and efficiency in the afternoon.

To put it another way, a good breakfast is *protective*. It will prevent you from being so famished by lunchtime that all your restraint vanishes and you overeat—and suffer the mind-numbing consequences afterward.

A particular client comes to mind in this context. A brilliant microbiologist, he came to me for help because he suspected he had a bizarre eating disorder. He explained that he entered the university cafeteria each day determined to eat only a mixed green salad and cottage cheese for lunch, but he *always* ended up with a tray piled high—with *two* cheeseburgers, French fries, and ice cream, pie, or cake.

When I asked him what he usually ate for breakfast, he looked at me as though I'd taken leave of my senses. "Why, just black coffee," was his answer. "I've always considered it positively uncivilized to eat first thing in the morning!"

I told him that if he couldn't force himself to eat real food—and not just coffee—before he left the house at seven, he should have a small breakfast snack in midmorning. A bagel and low-fat yogurt or an individual serving of dry cereal and low-fat milk from the vending machine in his department would take the edge off his hunger and make it easier for him to restrain himself at lunchtime. He followed my advice, and, I'm pleased to say, that was the end of the problem.

With a late breakfast snack, this scientist was eating in sync with his biological rhythms and thus deriving the benefits of entraining. He was able to control his food intake at noon. And he discovered that when he did not overeat at lunch, he could work smarter and harder throughout the afternoon, without the groggy sluggishness—a result of calorie over-load—that had cut into his afternoon productivity in the past.

Best Breakfast Bets

TIMING. Breakfast, in my definition, is simply the meal that comes before lunch. It is not necessary to eat immediately upon arising, but for maximum entraining you should get some food into your system within three hours of awakening. If you are a very early riser, however, and eat a very early breakfast, midmorning hunger—which can lead to overeating at lunch and a subsequent fall-off in afternoon performance—may be as big a problem for you as it was for my client who ate *no* breakfast. Just as judicious snacking helped him avoid lunch-time calorie overload and its inevitable consequence, post-meal performance dip, so will it help you. (Later in this chapter you will find a number of low-calorie morning snack suggestions that will take the edge off hunger and enable you to function at peak levels until lunch.)

WHAT AND HOW MUCH TO EAT. Breakfast should be rich in vitamins, minerals, and other essential nutrients but low in fat, too much of which can make you feel slowed-down or mud-dled, despite the fact that your biological cycles are all on the upswing.

A good breakfast should also supply enough calories to fuel your anticipated energy needs. No, you needn't get out your calculator, calorie counter, or energy expenditure chart to figure it all out. It isn't necessary to be *that* precise. Simply try to scale the size of your breakfast to *approximately* the amount of *physical* activity you plan to engage in that morning.

For example, if you jog, swim, or otherwise work out in the morning, or if your job or weekend recreation requires that you do a lot of heavy lifting, pushing, hammering, sawing, etc., you obviously will need more calories at breakfast than if you merely shower, dress, drive to the office, and then sit at a desk till lunch. Eat accordingly.

Seven Days of High-Power Breakfasts

The following weeks of breakfast menus will give you maximum entraining benefits if each meal is eaten within the first three or four hours after awakening. These meals will also fulfill your nutritional requirements and their calorie content is appropriate if your job is sedentary and you do not exercise early in the day.

Calorie Alert!

Menus here and throughout this book are all low in fat but not necessarily low in calories. If you are watching your weight but still want all the benefits of eating to manage your mind and your moods, decrease the portion sizes. Conversely, if you usually eat much more than I have recommended yet have no problem with weight gain, you may increase portion sizes so that your food intake corresponds more closely to what is normal for you.

MENU #1
1 fresh fruit (an apple, orange, peach, pear, etc.—or ½–¾ cup berries), sliced and mixed into
8 ounces plain yogurt
1 bran muffin, with 1–2 teaspoons jelly or diet margarine
Beverage as usual (use milk if desired, not cream)

MENU #2
4–6 ounces fruit juice (orange, grapefruit, cranberry)
1–2 scrambled eggs
1–2 slices whole-wheat toast topped with a slice of low-fat cheese, such as skim-milk mozzarella
Beverage as usual (use milk if desired, not cream)

MENU #3

4–6 ounces fruit juice (orange, grapefruit, cranberry)
1–1½ cups hot cereal (such as oatmeal or Wheatena), topped with
Sliced banana
Beverage as usual (use milk if desired, not cream)

MENU #4

4–6 ounces fruit juice (orange, grapefruit, cranberry)
1–2 slices French toast (use commercial frozen variety if time is
    short), topped with
½ cup cottage cheese with pineapple
Beverage as usual (use milk if desired, not cream)

MENU #5

4–6 ounces fruit juice (orange, grapefruit, cranberry)
8 ounces plain, lemon, or vanilla-flavored yogurt, sprinkled with
½ cup granola and 2 tablespoons raisins, chopped dates, or dried
    apricots
Beverage as usual (use milk if desired, not cream)

MENU #6

1 fresh fruit (grapefruit, orange, peach, pear, apple—or ½–¾ cup
    berries)
1 bagel, topped with
¼ cup ricotta cheese and 1 slice lox if desired *or* 1–2 slices melted
    mozzarella cheese
Beverage as usual (use milk if desired, not cream)

MENU #7

4–6 ounces fruit juice (orange, grapefruit, cranberry)
1½ cups high-fiber cold cereal, topped with
½ cup berries *or* ½ sliced banana
½ cup low-fat milk
Beverage as usual (use milk if desired, not cream)

Breakfasts to Avoid

As I mentioned earlier, fat, though it neither increases nor decreases production of the mind- and mood-modifying brain chemicals, has little or no place in a power breakfast. *It is hardly ever a good choice at any meal.* Fat delivers more calories per gram (9) than any other nutrient, so it is always to be avoided if your goal is either to lose pounds or maintain your weight.

More to the point here, however, is the fact that, as mentioned earlier, high-fat foods take so long to digest. And the longer digestion takes, the more blood is diverted to the intestinal tract, where the complicated process of turning food into its useable nutritional components takes place. Although we still do not know exactly why, when blood is diverted down to your stomach and intestines rather than up to your brain, mental energy and acuity tend to diminish.

Thus high-fat foods head the list of breakfast items *not* to eat. You probably already know most of the high-fat foods by heart, but they are worth listing again.

Avoid these breakfast foods:

- Sausages, bacon, or even ham (unless it is very lean)
- French fries, greasy home fries, and hash-browned potatoes
- Cream cheese or butter. (Try low-fat ricotta or low-fat chive-flavored cottage cheese on toast or bagels instead. Delicious!)
- Fast-food combos such as sausage-and-egg croissants, ham-and-cheese croissants, and English muffins topped with cheese, egg, and sausage
- Eggs Benedict, eggs Mornay, or any eggs or omelette made with a rich cheesy or creamy sauce
- "Farmers' breakfasts" (those "three eggs, plus bacon or ham plus hash-brown potatoes plus heavily buttered toast" extravaganzas advertised in the Midwest)

- Pastries such as doughnuts, croissants, coffee cake, biscuits, sweet rolls, and Danishes

How to Choose the Best of the Worst

Let's imagine that you find yourself at breakfast time in a restaurant or coffee shop that serves few of the good things and specializes instead in the foods I have been urging you to avoid. Here's how to choose in order to do the least mental damage:

- Order a plain doughnut instead of one that is glazed, iced, or filled with chocolate or cream.
- Ask for a plain croissant with no butter rather than for the chocolate or cheese-filled variety.
- Choose a plain or cinnamon Danish in lieu of a cheese Danish. Better still, ask for toast or a bagel or bran muffin, and tell the waiter to hold the butter and cream cheese.
- Have a bran, corn, or English muffin instead of French fries, home fries, or hash browns.
- Keep in mind that a plain biscuit or croissant is better than one of the cheese and egg and/or bacon-filled fast-food biscuit specialties.
- If you are in the mood for an egg, have it poached or soft-boiled or scrambled in a tiny dab of butter or margarine rather than fried.
- Choose lean ham (or any ham, and trim away the fat yourself) instead of bacon or sausage.

Breakfasts for Stay-at-Homes

A problem for many men and women who work at home is that they are so busy making sure that children and spouse get off to a good start that they forget—or are too rushed—to sit down and have something nutritious for themselves. This is always a mistake. You, too, will benefit from the entraining effect of proper food in the morning. And remember the lunchtime trap you unwittingly set for yourself by not eating anything until the middle of the day, when hunger finally catches up with you. The overeating that results may make you feel too sluggish, slowed down, and sleepy to push on effectively during the hours that follow.

One of my clients, a school teacher, was puzzled by the changes that took place in her moods and her ability to function efficiently once summer vacation had started.

"I don't understand it," she said at her first visit to my office one day in late June. "As a first grade teacher instructing twenty-nine active children how to read, write, add, and subtract, I have to be alert every minute. I love it and I'm good at my job.

"Yet," she continued, "during the summer I can barely deal with my own two kids. After lunch, I feel like napping . . . but, of course, that's when the children want to go to the beach or the park. Yet I'm so tired and fuzzy-headed that I don't trust myself to drive."

When I asked about her eating habits, she told me that she *always* ate breakfast during the school year—usually cereal, milk, and fruit. But she purposely skipped the meal in summer because, as she put it, "I'm always around food when I'm in the house, and I don't want to gain weight. Cutting out breakfast seems like a good way to save calories."

"What about lunch?" I asked.

"Well," she responded, "I always fix a big one. I'm so hungry by the middle of the day that I usually follow my lunch with what the kids leave over from *their* lunch and then top it all off with ice cream and cookies."

My suggestion was simple: Start eating a low-fat breakfast and see what happens.

The next time she came to my office, in mid-July, she told me that she definitely felt better—more cheerful, energetic, effective, patient, and persistent in getting things done. Once she began to eat enough good, healthy food in the morning, her need for an enormous lunch disappeared, and so did her afternoon muddleheadedness. Her "winter personality" had returned.

Hurry-up Breakfast Tips

• If you simply cannot make time for a leisurely sit-down breakfast at home, you can stow most of the makings of the meals listed above in plastic containers in the fridge, then pop them into your briefcase or bag as you rush out the door.

• Or pick up breakfast items on the way to work. Most coffee shops, delis, and convenience stores stock fresh fruit, juices, muffins, single-serving packets of cereal, and containers of milk, cottage cheese, and yogurt. (In a pinch, you don't even need a spoon for your yogurt. I know a runner who drinks his yogurt after his morning workout. The trick is to shake the container vigorously—with top firmly in place, of course—until the yogurt liquefies.)

Midmorning Power Snacking

In many offices and other places of employment, a fifteen- or twenty-minute midmorning break is traditional. I suspect the custom originated many years ago when unions wanted to give assembly line and other laborers a much-needed respite from monotonous and/or physically strenuous work. If your job requires heavy physical labor, you probably will need something to eat between breakfast and lunch. But if your work requires brain rather than muscle power, a midmorning snack may do more harm than good.

If you have eaten an adequate breakfast, a midmorning snack will add unnecessarily to your daily calorie total—unless, of course, you compensate by eating a smaller lunch or dinner.

Worse, if you choose typical coffee break fare—a sweet roll, Danish, croissant, or other high-carb, high-fat, high-calorie pastry, for example—the result may be a mini-postmeal dip in mental alacrity and performance as your stomach and other digestive organs contend with the food.

For most mental workers, the best midmorning snack is no snack at all.

There are exceptions to every rule, of course, and the exceptions to this one have to do with what you ate for breakfast, and when you ate it.

As I explained earlier in this chapter, a good breakfast is important. But if circumstances or your own lack of appetite first thing in the morning make it impossible for you to eat a real breakfast at the customary breakfast hour, you *should* have something nourishing at midmorning to tide you over until lunch. Or, if you awaken *very* early and eat breakfast immediately upon arising, as many dynamic overachievers who can't wait to get on with the day's work often do, you will no doubt be hungry and need something to eat by ten or so.

Non-breakfast eaters and very early breakfast eaters who try to make it all the way to lunch without a midmorning snack may be so hungry by noon that they overeat—and afterward feel too brain-drained and sluggish to function effectively.

To reiterate: If you eat an adequate breakfast at a normal hour, you won't need and shouldn't indulge in a midmorning snack.

Relax. Chat with coworkers and colleagues. Maybe even do a few minutes of light exercise (such as jogging in place, knee bends, or walking briskly around the block). Sip some fruit juice or ice water, or have a cup of coffee or tea, if you usually have a caffeinated beverage at this time. But don't eat.

However, if you had no breakfast or ate so early that you are beginning to feel hungry by midmorning, the following low-fat midmorning snack suggestions will see you through until lunch without adding drastically to your calorie total for the day or resulting in a mentally debilitating postmeal dip.

A.M. SNACK #1
4–6 ounces orange or grapefruit juice
2–3 rice cakes
1 slice low-fat cheese, such as skim-milk mozzarella

A.M. SNACK #2
8 ounces low-fat chocolate milk (made with skim milk)
1–2 slices raisin bread
2 teaspoons ricotta cheese

A.M. SNACK #3
1–2 ounces chicken, turkey, or tuna
1 slice bread or 3″ pita bread
1 medium carrot

A.M. SNACK #4
Low-cholesterol egg salad, made with 1 hard-boiled egg, 1 hard-boiled egg white, and 1 teaspoon diet mayonnaise, mixed with chopped celery if desired, on
1 roll

A.M. SNACK #5
4–6 ounces low-fat plain or pineapple-flavored cottage cheese on 1 corn or bran Toastee

Lunches with Punch

Lunch is a critical meal because it usually is eaten just at the point when the upward surge of morning mental and physical energy begins to level off.

The food you get into your system at midday can produce brain chemical changes that will sustain the alertness, zip, and responsiveness you felt earlier—or hasten the cyclical down-swing into lower levels of energy, attentiveness, and motivation.

Although I am not aware of any scientific studies that have focused specifically on the subject, I would venture to say that eating the wrong food at lunch is a major reason for afternoon procrastination.

Brain-Powering Lunch Strategies

The power eating strategy at breakfast is to synchronize food intake with rising biological cycles in order to give those cycles an extra boost upward. At lunch the goal is to keep those peaking cycles propped up as long as possible.

How can you do it? Part of the answer is revealed by your responses to the food/mind/mood tests you took in chapter 4. Look at your ratings after you ate the protein-based lunch. Now compare them with the way you felt after eating the carbohydrate-based lunch.

If you responded like the majority of our food/mind/mood volunteers, you felt like a tiger (well . . . almost) after the protein lunch. In any event, you were mentally sharper and more responsive than after your carbohydrate test lunch, which may have left you feeling more like a pussycat—slower, more relaxed, perhaps even ready for a short afternoon nap.

Now, there are times, such as weekends and vacations, when you might want to cultivate a luxuriously languorous state of mind and body after your midday meal. And when that is the case, I heartily recommend a substantial, high-carbohydrate meal, accompanied, perhaps, with a glass of excellent vintage wine.

But, unless your work involves demonstrating sleep sofas in a department store, a substantial high-carb meal is exactly what you should avoid on workdays—or on any day when you must stay alert and respond quickly and accurately to every mental challenge.

How to Pack More Power into Your Lunch

To prop up energy levels that are on the verge of sagging and to maintain mental alertness and motivation throughout the middle hours of the day, your lunch must be (1) high in protein, (2) both low in fat and relatively low in calories, and (3) alcohol-free.

Lunchtime protein is important. When your brain's supply of dopamine and norepinephrine is beginning to run short—as is often the case during and after periods of intense mental activity—the amino acid tyrosine, supplied by high-protein food, will be used by your brain to synthesize more of the two alertness chemicals.

Eating protein maintains mental sharpness indirectly as well, because the flood of amino acids supplied by high-protein foods prevents your brain from manufacturing serotonin, the calming chemical. Thus, even when your brain's supply of norepinephrine and dopamine is ample and eating more protein won't stimulate greater production of the two alertness chemicals, it will inhibit the manufacture of serotonin. This means that you are less likely to experience the slowed-down, more passive, and relaxed state of mind that occurs when serotonin is produced.

Later in the day you may want and even need the calming, focusing effects of carbohydrate, and I will tell you why and how to use these valuable foods when we get to the section on dinners. But for lunch you should concentrate on high-energy protein foods. (See the menu suggestions that follow.)

Workday lunches should be low in fat and calories. Remember, fat takes longer to digest than other nutrients and leaves less blood available to other organ systems and cells, including those in your brain. So mental energy tends to ebb after a high-fat meal. And of course, there are all those calories . . .

If you want to keep your brain powered throughout the afternoon, the light lunch is the right lunch.

Avoid alcohol. Even if alcohol didn't have a mind-muddling effect of its own, I would still advise you to drink nothing stronger than coffee, tea, soda, or seltzer with your midday meal. Not that I expect you to walk the straight and narrow path of total abstinence. I think wine, beer, and cocktails in moderation are wonderful at the right time and in the right place. But workday lunches are neither the time nor place to enjoy them.

Not only will alcoholic beverages slow you down, they may make you forget to eat the right things.

One of the characteristics people most like about alcohol is its capacity for relaxing inhibitions. And once inhibitions are reduced enough, your resolve to eat a high-energy, high-protein, low-fat lunch can easily melt away.

WHAT AND HOW MUCH TO EAT. How *much* do you need at lunch to maintain your high-level state of mental alertness after lunch? Follow these general guidelines:

- Have between three and five ounces of meat, poultry, seafood, or fish (tuna and sardines count as fish, of course) *or*
- Approximately one cup (eight ounces) of low-fat yogurt or cottage cheese *or*
- Two ounces of cheese, such as low-fat mozzarella, ricotta, or feta *or*
- Two eggs. (However, because of their very high cholesterol content, you should have no more than three or four "visible" eggs per week.)

Seven Days of Brain-Powering Lunches

The menus that follow represent a week's worth of lunches, all high in protein, low in fat, and relatively low in calories (although none of them are diet lunches *per se*). They are the lunches of choice for afternoon peak performance.

MENU #1

3 ounces tuna mixed with chopped chives, scallions, celery, and
   drizzled with lemon juice and 1 teaspoon olive oil (or 1 tablespoon diet mayonnaise) on
2 slices of whole-grain bread
4 ounces lettuce, raw broccoli, and carrot salad with
1–2 teaspoons oil and vinegar or low-calorie dressing
8 ounces low-fat milk

MENU #2

Greek salad with 3–5 ounces feta cheese. (Ask the waiter or
   waitress to serve dressing on the side; drizzle on 1 or 2 teaspoons.)
6″ pita bread
1 cup fresh fruit salad or 1 piece fruit
8 ounces low-fat milk

MENU #3

3–4 ounces lean roast beef
2 slices whole-grain bread, a bagel, or a roll
1 sliced tomato
3/4 cup sherbet
8 ounces low-fat milk

MENU #4

1 cup low-fat cottage cheese, mixed with
1 sliced peach, pear, or pineapple or 3/4 cup berries
1 whole-grain roll or corn or bran muffin
8 ounces low-fat milk

MENU #5

3–4 ounces sliced chicken (with skin removed)
2 slices whole-grain bread, roll, or pita bread. (Spread with
   mustard or ketchup if desired, or 1 teaspoon mayonnaise or 1
   tablespoon diet mayonnaise.)
1 apple, pear, or other fruit
8 ounces low-fat milk

MENU #6
1½ cups chili*
1 cup raw cauliflowerets, cucumber, broccoli, and/or carrots
1 package saltines
8 ounces low-fat milk

MENU #7
2 sliced hard-boiled eggs on
2 slices whole-grain bread, spread with 2 teaspoons mayonnaise
    (or 1 tablespoon diet mayonnaise), if desired
1 cup mixed green salad with tomato wedges and 1–2 teaspoons
    Italian dressing*
1 apple or banana
8 ounces low-fat milk

Common Lunchtime Fat Traps and How to Avoid Them

I have said it before and will probably make the point many times again throughout this book: High-fat, high-calorie foods get in the way of clear, creative thinking and peak mental performance.

Surprisingly, many of my most nutritionally sophisticated patients are not aware of how much fat they consume, because it is often a hidden ingredient in dishes we tend to think of as being low-calorie.

A svelte young personnel manager of a downtown Boston bank, for example, told me that she adored Mexican food, and all the more because "it's so low in fat." Thinking of the non-fried flour tortillas topped with small amounts of shredded chicken or beef, lettuce, and tomato, I agreed. In fact, I encouraged her to eat such food—but to avoid the cheese and sour cream that is sometimes served along with it.

*See recipe in Appendix B.

It seems we were talking at cross purposes.

"Oh, but I *never* eat tortillas," she said. "They're so fattening, aren't they? Instead I order taco chips and guacamole dip, which is, after all, just a mashed-up vegetable."

Taco chips are fried and contain quite a bit of fat. As for the guacamole, it is made from a fruit—the avocado—and it is a fruit with a *very* high fat content. My patient's idea of low-fat eating was clearly off base.

And then there was the sales executive who told me with obvious pride that he always went to a salad bar for lunch because "a salad is a light, low-fat meal."

Curious, I asked him what kind of salads he favored. He told me he started out with a bed of lettuce . . . so far so good. But then he went on to say that he usually added a scoop of potato salad and then a scoop of macaroni salad and sprinkled them both with bacon bits and grated cheese. "But the best part," he said, "is the blue cheese dressing. I'm very partial to it. I always leave lots of room in the bowl for it. And sometimes I dip my bread into the dressing instead of using butter."

I pointed out to him that his salad selections—potato salad and macaroni salad—both had mayonnaise as a major ingredient, and mayonnaise is almost as high in fat as butter. The bacon bits, cheese topping, and blue cheese dressing were also loaded with fat. We decided that he should stay away from the chic salad bar and settle for clear soup and a chicken sandwich with lettuce on rye at the old-fashioned luncheonette on the corner.

Here are common fat traps you should learn to avoid:

- Creamy soups and chowders. (Manhattan-style chowder, made with a tomato-based stock, is okay.)
- Fast-food hamburgers topped with bacon, cheese, and a mayonnaise-style sauce. When you must eat in a fast-food restaurant, have it your way, *without* all the extras on your burger.

- Batter-dipped then fried vegetables, such as zucchini, broccoli, cauliflower, onions. All of these are good, nutritious foods, but the batter coating and deep-frying make them too fatty and unsuitable for a power eating program.
- Baked potatoes and potato skins that are sprinkled with cheese or bacon or smothered in sour cream
- Fatty salad ingredients such as avocados, anchovies, bacon—and, of course, salad dressing, including French, Russian, blue cheese, creamy Italian, mayonnaise, and oil and vinegar (although vinegar or lemon alone would be just fine). A *small* amount of any dressing is permissible (a teaspoon or so), but too much can throw your mind- and mood-managing regimen off for the rest of the day. Limit amounts to one to two teaspoons.

Help! You're a Captive in an Ethnic Restaurant

Sooner or later—perhaps *often,* if your job requires frequent mixing of business with pleasure over lunch—you will find yourself in situations that allow you less control than usual over your food intake. This is frequently the case when you are invited to lunch in an ethnic or specialty restaurant. However, with the following guidelines in mind, you can keep your brain powered throughout the afternoon, even when you are confronted with a menu from which most of our recommended foods are conspicuously absent.

CHINESE RESTAURANTS. Delectable but bad from a lunchtime mind- and mood-managing point of view are dishes in which noodles or rice predominate. However, a small portion of rice—no more than ¾ cup—is harmless if you eat it with fish, shrimp, or other protein. Fish, shrimp, lobster, or chicken dishes featuring Chinese vegetables such as snow peas and water chestnuts are good choices. So are sautéed or stir-fried beef, since these cooking methods add only small amounts of fat and the red meat preferred in Chinese cookery tends to be very lean.

JAPANESE RESTAURANTS. Sushi, sashimi, and broiled fish or other seafood are practically made to order for power eaters, as are the many tofu-based Japanese dishes. Augment with steamed or stir-fried nonstarchy vegetables. Limit rice to ½ to ¾ cup. And, of course, *avoid* deep-fat fried tempura-style seafood and vegetables.

ITALIAN RESTAURANTS. Pasta freaks definitely should try to avoid spaghetti emporiums at lunchtime. Should you find yourself in the local trattoria at midday, don't even look at the pasta side of the menu, and close your eyes to the pork and sausage specialties. Instead, order poultry, broiled if available (trim away skin before eating), or veal, provided it is unbreaded and has no cheese coating. Better still, ask for a big salad of Italian greens, fava beans, Italian tuna, and plum tomatoes, with slices of skim-milk mozzarella, and have that with unbuttered Italian bread. Tell the waiter you want oil and vinegar *on the side*. If you *must* have pasta, order it as a side dish and eat it along with the protein entrée and not as an appetizer.

FRENCH RESTAURANTS. With the advent a few years ago of nouvelle cuisine (a revolutionary development in French cookery, featuring skimpy portions of light, exquisitely fresh food served without thick, buttery sauces), dining *à la Française* has become less damaging to postlunch performance than in the past. However, nouvelle cuisine is "out" now at some of the trendier French restaurants, and the classic heavily sauced style is back in. Skip the terrines, the pâtés, the filled puff-pastry appetizers, and anything that is blanketed with sauce beurre, Bearnaise, Mornay, or Hollandaise (especially Hollandaise). Instead, order plain fish or poultry; steamed, herbed but unbuttered and unsauced vegetables; a small boiled or baked potato or small portion of rice; and a salad with dressing on the side.

HEALTH FOOD RESTAURANTS. These usually small, very appealing places are almost by definition "meatless." That means that in order to get a good, high-protein lunch you will have to order something like a chopped-egg platter; tofu (soybean curd) in one form or another—but not fried; a dish featuring a low-fat cheese, such as skim-milk ricotta or mozzarella, or yogurt; or plain baked or grilled fish or regular water-packed tuna if available. Peanut butter and other nut or seed butters often included on health food menus contain protein but are so high in fat that a sandwich made with them may result in a postmeal dip in mental energy and motivation.

From Health Food Failure to Health Food Overachiever

My attitude toward health food is ambiguous. Most of it *is* healthy, but it won't help you manage your mind and mood unless you know what kind to eat, as well as when and under what circumstances.

The point was brought home to me by a client who was an art history major and spent much of each afternoon looking at slides in darkened lecture halls. She came to me distraught, actually considering changing her major because she was having such difficulty keeping herself awake after lunch. "As soon as the lights go out, so does my mind," she said.

As I soon learned, she was a quasi-vegetarian who avoided meat and poultry and lived mainly on fresh or canned fish, whole-grain breads, salads, and casseroles made from rice, beans, and/or peas.

Her usual lunch, which she either made at home or bought from a local health food store, consisted of two slabs of whole-grain bread spread with sesame seed butter, or a salad called

Lunches of Last Resort

There are two items available in every restaurant, diner, coffee shop, and other eatery in America. When in doubt about what to order, you can always rely on one of these as the basis of a high-protein, low-fat, and relatively low-calorie lunch that will stem the precipitous slide into mental lethargy during the afternoon. They are:

• *The hamburger.* But of course! Order a side dish of coleslaw instead of greasy French fries, and see if you can get the waiter or waitress to bring you a few tomato slices as well. Eat the smallest size plain hamburger on a roll, as a sandwich. Finish your meal with a glass of skim or low-fat milk.

• *The mixed green salad plus . . .* In most restaurants a chef's salad is listed on the menu. If so, order it, but tell the waiter to ask the cook to substitute tuna and/or lean beef, chicken, cottage, or feta cheese for the bologna, ham loaf, and Swiss or American cheese that are ingredients in the typical chef's salad. This substitution may cost you a dollar or so more, but it will also add hours of more productive, creative thinking to the rest of your day. Ask for oil and vinegar, rather than house dressing, and go light on the oil.

If there is no chef's salad on the menu, ask for a mixed green salad and request a few slices of chicken or roast beef or an individual-size can of water-packed tuna to go with it. Eat it with a roll, pita bread, or a muffin. Again, you will pay more than for a plain mixed green salad, but again, it will be worth it.

taboullah, made of bulgur wheat, tomatoes, and parsley, which she ate with a bran muffin and apple juice. Although these certainly are *healthy* lunches, in that they supply many important nutrients, they are also textbook examples of low-protein, high-carbohydrate meals.

My recommendations: Eat sandwiches made with thinly sliced whole-grain bread and tuna, low-fat ricotta cheese, or chopped egg. On days when she preferred a salad, she was to eat three or four ounces of tofu or low-fat cheese along with it. Instead of apple juice, I suggested she switch to skim milk.

I must admit that even I could hardly believe the incredible difference these high-protein meals made in her performance and behavior. No more fighting to stay awake in her afternoon classes. No more thoughts of changing her major. Suddenly she was all eager eyes and ears during lectures, able to take better organized and more detailed and coherent notes than ever before in her academic career. And all because of a few ounces of protein eaten at midday!

Afternoon Snacking—Who Needs It?

My advice to clients and to you about midafternoon snacking is much the same as for midmorning snacks: If you ate a good, nutritious lunch similar to those suggested earlier in this chapter, you probably won't *need* to eat anything at three or four in the afternoon. Your lunch supplied enough of the food energy you need to continue working smart with a high degree of mental alertness and productivity and without the distraction of hunger pangs.

Of course, I am assuming here that you will eat dinner somewhere between six-thirty and eight in the evening. On days when you will be starting your evening meal much later than that, you may well need something low in fat and low in calories to quiet the rumbling of your stomach and prevent the weakness and/or dizziness that sometimes occur when too many hours elapse between meals.

For most people, most of the time, a midafternoon break is better used for relaxation or to clear the mind with a few moments of fresh air and exercise than as an opportunity to eat. (Remember, we are concerned with routine days here. On days that demand more from you mentally, you may need the mind-powering, mood-enhancing benefit of certain foods in the afternoon. I will be telling you what to eat, why, and under which circumstances in the chapters that follow.)

For Carbohydrate Cravers Only: The Restorative Snack

Although I urge most of my clients not to snack in the afternoon on days that are only normally challenging, *some* men and women must snack or they run out of mental steam well before the workday has ended. Or they become too fidgety and restless to concentrate. Or they turn grouchy or irritable. Or they simply feel blah.

These are the people I call carbohydrate cravers.

How do you know if you are one of them? Take another look at the results of the food/mind/mood test given in chapter 4 to help you pinpoint your state of mind before and after eating a midafternoon carbohydrate snack.

You probably are *not* a carbohydrate craver if:

- You rated yourself as feeling somewhat or very energetic, motivated, and alert *both before and after* a carbohydrate snack.
- You rated yourself as feeling irritable, agitated, or sluggish and apathetic both *before and after* a carbohydrate snack.

But if you felt irritable, agitated, or sluggish and apathetic before a carbohydrate snack and then, an hour later, rated your state of mind as being more alert, vigorous, and motivated and/or calmer, more patient, and focused, it is a safe bet that you *are* a carbohydrate craver.

Carbohydrate cravers are not in the majority. Nevertheless, I have counseled many who were clients at the M.I.T. Research Center, and many more in my private practice.

Why should they be any different from other people? Why should you, if you are a carbohydrate craver, experience a decrease in your ability to work smart and perform efficiently, when others around you continue to function effortlessly and seemingly with mental energy to spare? These are questions that continue to puzzle me and other scientists with a special interest in the effects of food on mind and mood.

Although we do not know *why* some people are carbohydrate cravers and others are not, we have theories about the *cause* of food-related shifts in mood and state of mind. In people who are not carbohydrate cravers, serotonin levels tend to remain more or less constant during the day. It may be that in carbohydrate cravers serotonin levels drop off in the afternoon. However, it may not happen every day, and the state-of-mind changes may be very subtle in some people and quite pronounced in others.

We *do* know how to bring serotonin levels back up again, and that is by getting carbohydrate into the body and stimulating increased production of serotonin in the brain. For carbohydrate cravers, a sweet or starchy midafternoon snack can make an enormous difference!

There was, for example, the public health professional involved in a study of nutritional habits of thousands of subjects. Her job requires meticulous attention to detail, but when she came to me, she complained that her attention wandered in the afternoons, and she became so fidgety she found it difficult to work and took every opportunity to leave her desk. "I get hardly anything done after three o'clock, and the result is that there is that much more work to catch up on the following morning," she said.

And then there was the author who, despite deadline pressures, said that boredom and restlessness made it impossible for him to produce in the afternoon. "I'm a morning person," he told me. "The creative juices cease to flow later in the day. But I can't afford to throw my afternoons away and write only part-time."

For both of them, and for many others who came to me suspecting there might be a nutritional "cure" for afternoon slump, one to one and a half ounces of a starchy or sweet food made it possible to maintain brain power, motivation, and mental energy throughout the day!

Midafternoon Snacks for Carbohydrate Cravers

The snacks that are best for restoring mental energy and motivation, as well as for putting you back into a calmer, more relaxed, and focused state of mind, are sweets and starches in their purest form, unmixed with protein or fat. Good examples are the seven snack suggestions that follow.

One to one and a half ounces (30–45 grams) is the proper "dosage." However, people who are significantly overweight and women in the days just before a period may need to consume two to two and one-half ounces to get results. (But they should be sure to take the extra calories into account in managing their overall daily food plan.)

Eat carbohydrate snacks in the afternoon as needed—i.e., when you feel yourself sliding into a mental slump. It will pull you up and out again within half an hour or less!

SNACK #1
5 graham crackers or 15 Ritz crackers

SNACK #2
2-ounce package of Chuckles or 15 jelly beans

SNACK #3
1 English, bran, or corn muffin with 1 teaspoon jelly

SNACK #4
1½ ounces caramel-coated popcorn or 1½ ounces Cracker Jacks

SNACK #5
2 chocolate-covered vanilla ice cream bars on a stick or 2 Fudgsicles

SNACK #6
1½ cups Cheerios, Sugar Crisp, or Apple Jacks cereal without milk

SNACK #7
2 bars Pillsbury Fudge Jumble or a 1.7-ounce Pepperidge Farm Snack Bar

Dinners That Do What You Want Them to Do

Dinner, the last major meal of the day, is normally served at a time when the complex biological cycles that govern mental and physical energy are beginning to wind down. This easing off at the end of the day is neither good nor bad. It's simply fact.

It is also fact that you can use the food you eat at dinner to manage the way you feel and perform in the hours before you turn in for the night, either countering your circadian rhythms or enhancing them. You can make dinner a meal that literally will add to the number of productive hours in your day by helping you stay alert and mentally active well past your normal "closing time." Or you can choose food that will work *with* your biological rhythms, easing you into a more relaxed, unstressed state of mind and readying you for a refreshing night's sleep.

Dinners That Will Keep You Going

Everyone deserves and needs to relax at some point in the day, and for most people the period following dinner, when biological cycles are shifting into a presleep mode, is the ideal time for taking it easy.

However, for many active men and women the dinner hour is just a brief respite between daytime responsibilities and evening obligations. You may be one of them. Your job, for example, may require that you take work home from the office more or less regularly. Or perhaps you attend evening classes. Or you may be involved in volunteer activities or belong to an amateur drama group or singing society. Or maybe the time between dinner and bed is the *only* open slot in your schedule for paying bills and balancing your checkbook, keeping up with personal correspondence, helping the kids with their homework, and reading journals and publications related to your job.

Or, like millions of others, it could be that you simply *want* to be able to use after-dinner time more productively.

The question is, do you have the mental energy to accomplish all that you must or would like to do? If your answer is "usually not," you certainly are not alone. The late-day winding down of mind and body is a universal phenomenon, although obviously some people wind down more quickly and completely than others.

A large evening meal hastens biological slowdown. If you want to maintain high mental performance levels after dinner, remember your brain power and mental energy are always diminished by overeating, but never more dramatically than in the evening. The more you consume at dinner, the more you will long for your bed and not your briefcase.

If your goal is to continue to be productive after your evening meal but you frequently feel brain-drained or too mentally muddled to carry on, it may very well be because you are overloading your stomach.

However, I know from clinical experience with clients and from working with them in my private practice that simply prescribing fewer calories isn't enough to counter biological slowdown and reenergize the mind.

Too many high-carbohydrate, low-protein foods at dinner will put you to sleep. Carbohydrates, which stimulate your brain to make more of the calming chemical, serotonin, *always* tend to create a more relaxed state of mind. But late in the day, when biological rhythms are slowing, readying you for sleep, high-carbohydrate foods enhance feelings of drowsiness.

Proteins, on the other hand, act to prevent serotonin production, especially when they are eaten before or with carbohydrates. Remember, the amino acids in protein also encourage the brain to make more of the alertness chemicals, dopamine and norepinephrine.

Eating for mental energy in the evening requires that you keep calories low by limiting fat and portion sizes, and that you get protein into your system before or along with carbohydrates.

The following meals to stay alert by are all relatively high in protein, supply only moderate amounts of carbohydrates, and are small enough and low enough in fat not to promote postmeal dip. Keep in mind, when you sit down to eat, that it is important *not to begin your meal with carbohydrates*. Your first few bites should be of protein; then you can proceed to the starchy component of your dinner.

Seven Days of Energizing Dinners

These meals probably are smaller than those you are accustomed to eating, in which case you may leave the table feeling somewhat less than completely sated. Good! The feelings of fullness that you experience after larger, more calorific meals are partly responsible for decreased brain power and mental energy later on in the evening. When you have finished one of the following dinners and are deeply immersed in your chosen evening's activity, whatever it may be, I promise you won't feel hungry. You will be too busy accomplishing what you want to do.

MENU #1
5–6 ounces broiled or poached fish
1–1½ cups steamed julienne carrots, fennel, and leeks
3 boiled new potatoes
1 cup spinach salad with 1–2 teaspoons Italian dressing*
1 wedge cantaloupe or other melon

MENU #2
4–5 ounces veal *tonnato**
½ cup steamed green beans
1 medium oven-roasted potato, with no dressing
3 slices *fresh* pineapple

MENU #3
4–5 ounces broiled, skinned boneless chicken
1 cup stir-fried mixed vegetables (broccoli, water chestnuts, onions, etc.)
¾ cup steamed rice
1 fresh orange, sliced

MENU #4
4–5 ounces Chinese pot roast*
¾ cup steamed vegetables (carrots, snow peas, celery, etc.)
¾ cup Chinese noodles
¾ cup sliced strawberries

MENU #5
1½ cups Creole fish chowder*
1 cup spinach salad
1 poached pear

MENU #6
1 serving stuffed cabbage rolls*
¾ cup poached egg noodles
¾ cup salad made of mixed fresh fruit

*See recipe in Appendix B.

MENU #7
4–5 ounces roast London broil*
3/4 cup steamed turnips
1 cup green beans
1/2–3/4 cup couscous or rice
1 medium baked apple

Dinners for When You Want to Unwind

Now let's say you've been working hard all day and have no particular plans for after dinner other than to spend a quiet time with friends or family, perhaps watch some television, or read for the sheer enjoyment of it (as opposed to studying work- or school-related material). What should you have for dinner when your goal is simply to relax and unwind after an active, pressure-filled day?

Under these circumstances, what and how much you eat should be dictated solely by nutritional and caloric considerations. In other words, your evening meal should be healthy, well-balanced, and not cause your calorie total for the day to shoot up like a rocket. Eat slowly in a calm, stress-free atmosphere if possible. If a glass or two of wine with your meal helps you relax, so much the better.

With no mentally taxing demands on your evening agenda, you can savor your dinner and your digestive processes while the normal, natural end-of-day slowing of your biological rhythms do the rest.

Portion sizes are not given for the dinners suggested below because their calming properties do not depend on your eating the various foods in any particular amount. Be guided by your own sense of how much is enough, and then stop.

MENU #1
Pasta with seafood and mushroom sauce*
Asparagus
Melon

*See recipe in Appendix B.

MENU #2
White bean soup*
Mixed green salad
Cornbread
Blueberries

MENU #3
Meat-filled tortellini (can be bought ready-made)
Salad of tomato, red pepper, mozzarella, and greens, with oil and
    vinegar dressing as desired
Italian bread
Sorbet

MENU #4
Beef stew*
Carrot and cabbage salad
Sliced peaches and strawberries

MENU #5
Linguine with shrimp sauce*
Roast red pepper and mushroom salad
Garlic bread
Italian ices

MENU #6
Potato salad with chopped egg and tuna*
Coleslaw
Pumpernickel bread
Grapefruit and orange segments

MENU #7
Chicken Morocco*
Lettuce and tomato salad
French bread
Kiwi fruit

*See recipe in Appendix B.

Snacks to Sleep By

Your biological rhythms are programmed to shift down into a sleep mode at about the same time each evening. Sleep remains a mystery to science, but it is thought that a hormone called melatonin and several brain chemicals—including serotonin—are involved in inducing sleep and sustaining it throughout the night.

Eating foods that encourage your brain to manufacture more serotonin will ease the transition from wakefulness to sleep, gently nudging you over the threshold of drowsiness and into slumber.

The serotonin-producing foods, of course, are carbohydrates.

If sleep comes easily, you won't need a bedtime snack. It will only add calories to your daily total, and if you eat too much of the wrong kinds of food, it might actually interfere with your ability to drift off into slumber. (In chapter 11 I will tell you how to use certain foods to stay awake and remain mentally productive throughout the night.)

But if you have problems in going quickly and easily to sleep, you really cannot do better than to have one to one and a half ounces of a sweet or starch at bedtime. For most people, this is as effective as a sleeping pill, but without the side effect of morning grogginess and the potential for abuse inherent in sleep drugs.

Carbohydrate works even for dynamic, intense individuals whose brains never seem to stop whirring. It works even when the user is skeptical.

I have one client, for example, an extremely successful, hard-driving executive who is so focused on his job that when he gets into bed at night he commonly finds himself unable to stop replaying the accomplishments of that day and projecting ahead to all he intends to achieve the following day. Until he took advantage of a bedtime carbohydrate snack, he said, it seemed to take him ages to fall asleep.

I prescribed the usual dose of one to one and a half ounces of carbohydrate, to be taken approximately thirty minutes before he wanted to fall asleep. He looked doubtful. Why should eating carbohydrate work when hot baths, reading a boring book, counting sheep, drinking warm milk, and every other measure he had tried didn't slow the spinning of his mind? Nevertheless, he agreed to give bedtime carbohydrate a try. Next time I saw him, he was a true believer!

Seven Sleep-Inducing Bedtime Snacks

The best carbohydrate snacks—those that provide the quickest, surest results—are low in fat and contain very little or no protein. Low fat content keeps calories under control and avoids problems as a result of fat's being slow to digest. (In fact, the activity in your stomach after you eat a high-fat snack may prolong sleeplessness.) As for protein, you already know that it interferes with serotonin production by blocking access to the brain of the amino acid tryptophan. Thus protein, too, can keep you awake.

Milk, incidentally, is a protein food, and whole milk is fairly high in fat, which is why—despite its reputation for being a good food for wooing sleep—drinking milk at bedtime so rarely produces the desired results. Even a little milk poured on cereal can diminish the effectiveness of this excellent bedtime carbohydrate. If you don't want to eat cereal dry, do as another of my clients does; make hot instant cereal with boiling water, then sweeten it with one or two teaspoons of brown sugar or honey. It works so well that after eating his cereal, this client is often too sleepy even to rinse out his bowl!

BEDTIME SNACK #1
1 blueberry or corn Toastee

BEDTIME SNACK #2
1½ cups of any breakfast cereal (without milk)

BEDTIME SNACK #3
1½ ounces caramel-coated popcorn

BEDTIME SNACK #4
8 Social Tea biscuits or 3 fig bars or 6 ginger snaps

BEDTIME SNACK #5
1 cinnamon-raisin English muffin

BEDTIME SNACK #6
1 ⅝-ounce package of cinnamon and spice instant oatmeal (Harvest brand) *or*
1½ ounces maple and brown sugar instant oatmeal (H-O brand)

BEDTIME SNACK #7
1 toaster-size frozen waffle, spread with 1 tablespoon maple syrup

A Few Words About
Measuring Your Food

Throughout this morning-to-midnight power eating guide, I have been specific with regard to the number of cups or ounces of various foods to eat in order to obtain the maximum benefits of the food/mind/mood response.

Measuring should be no problem when you are at home. No doubt your kitchen is equipped with a measuring cup; you probably have a food scale, too. If you don't own the latter, consider buying one. A food scale doesn't cost much, and it will be worth every cent you pay for it, because with one of these gadgets on hand, you always will be able to prepare and serve food in amounts that are best for you.

Having a food scale will help you indirectly when you eat in a restaurant or at someone else's home. After the third or fourth time you have weighed and served yourself a six-ounce portion of fish at home, for example, you will have a good idea of what six ounces of fish look like, and you will be able to judge by eye how much to eat when you dine out. (The same is true, of course, of all the other foods you measure and weigh at home.)

Another way to accustom your eye to correct portion sizes of protein foods is to spend time in a supermarket, noting the weights of various packaged cuts of meat, poultry, fish, etc.

When in doubt about how much protein to eat, keep in mind that even lean beef and veal contain somewhat more fat than chicken or turkey (without the skin) or fish and other seafood. Since fat is *always* to be avoided when you want to manage your mind and your moods with food, it is best to err on the side of eating a little *less* beef or veal than your best estimate of what is appropriate. You have more leeway with the other proteins. Assuming that chicken, turkey, and seafood have been cooked without fat, you can safely eat a little more and still obtain good results with these food/mind/mood strategies.

The eating guidelines in this chapter will help you power your brain and maximize your performance all day and every day. Use them to give yourself an almost-instant boost in mental energy, to focus your thoughts, to work smarter in the morning and afternoon, to combat brain drain in the evening, and, at the end of the day, to get to sleep safely and surely. I know the results will be as gratifying to you as they have been to my clients.

6. Caffeine:
A Mind- and
Mood-Boosting Plus

Practically all the experts are telling you to cut back on caffeine. Soft drink companies and the makers of over-the-counter pain-killers base entire ad campaigns on the fact that their products are caffeine-free.

Caffeine is controversial at the moment, but the hard truth of the matter is this: There is very little scientific evidence that drinking coffee and other caffeine-containing beverages *in moderation* will have harmful long-term effects on health. The key phrase, of course, is *in moderation*. I'm not going to urge you to drink pots and pots of strong coffee or tea, because it isn't necessary. Very small amounts of caffeine are all you need to reap its benefits.

Nevertheless, the cons of caffeine need to be discussed, and I will get to them later in this chapter. For now, let's look at the pros.

Caffeine is a mind-accelerating mood booster. This isn't just sales hype brewed up by the coffee industry; it is scientific fact.

Most coffee drinkers are aware that their favorite beverage has a beneficial effect on their mental processes, especially coffee drunk first thing in the morning. As a client of mine so aptly put it, "That first cup of the day seems to clear the cobwebs from the brain." Now the effects of caffeine on cerebral activity has been documented.

The Great M.I.T. Caffeine Test-In

Not long ago, Dr. Harris Lieberman, a psychologist at M.I.T., rounded up a group of volunteers for the purpose of testing the relation of caffeine to mental processes. Some of the volunteers were habitual heavy coffee drinkers; others rarely or never touched the stuff, nor did they use other caffeine-containing beverages, such as cola-type soft drinks.

The tests were carried out over a period of several days but were always scheduled for the early morning. Volunteers were instructed not to eat or drink anything from midnight the evening before. The idea, of course, was to duplicate as closely as possible the conditions under which most coffee drinkers take their first cup in the morning—but with one important exception.

To avoid the problem of volunteers attempting to guess whether they were getting "real" coffee or a decaffeinated brand—speculation that might have skewed the test results— Dr. Lieberman distributed caffeine in various dosages in pill form to some, while others got identical-looking but caffeine-free placebo pills. Thus, coffee drinkers and non-coffee drinkers alike were never sure whether the pills they took on any particular day contained caffeine, or if so, how much.

Shortly after swallowing their pills each morning, volunteers took part in tests similar to the ones I described in chapter 4. There were reaction-time tests that measured how quickly volunteers responded to sounds coming through earphones, for example. There were vigilance tests, in which volunteers listened for an hour to a series of tones, most of the same duration but a very few slightly shorter. (They had to depress a key when they heard the slightly shorter tones. In the entire sixty minutes of the test, the short tone comes up only eighteen times.)

There was also a paper and pencil test. In this one, volunteers were given a code in which symbols such as #, /, and ∧ each had a letter equivalent. The symbol #, for instance, might correspond to the letter *A*. A long series of letters was arranged in random order on a separate sheet of paper, and the volunteer had to enter the correct code symbol in a space beneath each letter. The test was set up in such a way that after ten years of use in various psychological studies, only one person ever had completed it totally successfully.

Caffeine improved mental performance on every one of these tests, as well as on others administered by Dr. Lieberman. (Similar results were obtained at a university lab in Switzerland and at the National Institutes of Health.) On the days when a volunteer took a caffeine pill, he or she consistently demonstrated increased reaction speed, better concentration, and greater accuracy than on caffeine-free placebo days.

I found the results of the one-hour vigilance test—in which short tones are interspersed with slightly shorter ones—especially interesting. Volunteers who had taken a caffeine pill remained alert and attentive to the end of the test. When those same volunteers were given a placebo, they became restless and bored. Some simply tuned out, and a few went to sleep.

Most important, from the mind- and mood-changing point of view of this book, however, is that caffeine had the same brain-powering effect on volunteers who were accustomed to drinking one, two, or more cups of coffee every morning as on those who *never* drank coffee or caffeinated beverages.

In other words, it wasn't habit. It wasn't the coffee drinker's anticipation of his or her morning "fix." Nor was it any special sensitivity to caffeine on the part of non-coffee drinkers that explained the dramatic test results.

It was the caffeine itself.

Caffeine's stimulating effect on brain and nervous system resulted in quicker thinking and reacting, greater alertness and accuracy, and extended attention spans on the part of volunteers after they had had their morning dose of this chemical.

How to Use Caffeine to Boost Morning Performance Levels

What coffee drinkers have known all along, and what tests such as Dr. Lieberman's have confirmed, is that caffeine can and does play an important role in elevating morning brain power. It is a role similar to that of the protein foods, which induce the brain to manufacture more of the alertness chemicals, dopamine and norepinephrine, although the metabolic processes that give you a mental lift after drinking coffee are quite different from the brain-chemistry changes caused by eating protein.

Why is caffeine especially valuable in the morning? The explanation has to do with the fact that brain cells are most sensitive to caffeine after many hours of abstinence and become somewhat less sensitive after consumption. Thus, your first cup of coffee—or tea—in the morning, when your system is relatively caffeine-free, gives you a more powerful jolt of alertness than that fourth cup at noon.

To start the day in top mental form, drink one or two cups of "real" (not decaffeinated) coffee soon after you get out of bed.

Perk it, drip it, or use instant if you prefer. Drink it black, or add low-fat milk or nondairy creamer. Sweeten it with a little sugar or saccharin. What you add or do not add to your coffee makes little difference except in terms of taste (and calories). The important thing is to get a moderate amount of caffeine into your system.

The caffeine effect will be noticeable within a matter of minutes, and it will continue to keep you alert and mentally energetic for many hours afterward.

The Afternoon Caffeine Pickup

Although many of my friends and colleagues who are almost constant coffee or tea drinkers have a hard time believing it, blood sampling and other biological tests indicate that caffeine level in the body remains high for several hours after the first cup or two in the morning.

This means that if you have your morning coffee or tea at about seven, the caffeine will continue to keep you more alert and more efficient for three, four, or even five or six hours, depending on how quickly your body metabolizes the chemical.

The mind- and mood-managing implications of caffeine's long-lasting effects are obvious.

If your body metabolizes caffeine relatively slowly, drinking more coffee or tea at traditional coffee-break time (around ten or ten-thirty in the morning) will *not* give an extra boost to your mental energy and performance, since your system then is still plentifully supplied with caffeine. Pouring more of the chemical into your body at that time is a little like attempting to make your car run better by stopping off for gas when the tank is almost full.

On the other hand, a cup of coffee drunk somewhere between three-thirty and four-thirty in the afternoon, when caffeine levels are significantly lower, will reawaken your brain and help power your mind for another six hours or so.

A well-known author of health and nutrition books, who also writes a column for a leading newspaper, tells me that after a single morning cup of coffee, she abstains entirely until about four o'clock. "That's when I really need it. How do I know? I begin to talk more slowly and write more slowly, and I need to think harder and longer for each new phrase. Then the coffee . . . My mind clears and I am able to get all the way through the rest of the workday, make dinner, and even do some additional writing at home early in the evening."

It can work for you, too.

If you go into a mental stall in the afternoon, get yourself back into mental gear by having a cup of coffee or tea along with a carbohydrate snack.

Why Caffeine and Carbohydrate Are a Perfect Afternoon Combination

Caffeine and carbohydrate together are a great team; they work synergistically to pull you up out of the typical afternoon slump, whether it manifests itself as distractibility and the fidgets, boredom, sluggishness, or just plain mind fatigue. One or two ounces of carbohydrate will stimulate your brain to produce serotonin, the calming chemical, which will help you settle down and refocus on the task at hand. Then the caffeine kicks in and pushes your mental energy up a few notches. And there you are, more composed, your powers of concentration restored and your brain clicking along again with greater speed and accuracy.

I don't think it is an accident that the elegant coffee houses that line the boulevards of every European city and the coffee shops proliferating on our own sidewalks and in shopping malls are thronged with customers in late afternoon. The popularity of an afternoon cup of coffee taken with a pastry or sweet is testimony to the mind-mending power combination of caffeine plus carbohydrates.

Evening Caffeine: Potential Costs, Possible Benefit

My recommendation with regard to getting more caffeine into your system after four-thirty or so in the afternoon is simple: *Avoid it.*

The effects of caffeine are long-lasting. The coffee that got you up and out of your late-afternoon slump will remain in your body for hours to come and, assuming you eat a sensible dinner similar to those suggested in chapter 5, your mental energy will be sustained until midevening.

Unless you metabolize caffeine very quickly, drinking coffee or any caffeinated beverage after dinner can interfere with your ability to relax, feel drowsy, and go to sleep at a reasonable hour. This is such common knowledge that I almost hesitate to put it down on paper. Yet, I am constantly amazed at the number of insomniacs who fail to make the connection between after-dinner coffee and the hours they spend tossing and turning in bed, waiting for sleep.

If you enjoy sipping something hot after your evening meal, the obvious choice is a decaffeinated coffee or tea. *Tip:* Some decaffeinated espressos are so rich in flavor that it is hard to believe they're not the real thing.

Of course, if you must stay awake much later than usual—in order to finish a report, for example—then after-dinner coffee or tea certainly can help to ward off sleepiness. But don't expect a renewed surge of mental energy and motivation after drinking a caffeinated beverage late in the day. The natural, biological tendency of your body after darkness arrives is to slow down and prepare for sleep. Caffeine will keep you from unwinding completely, but it won't wind you up to morning levels of alertness.

But Is It a Must?

Now that you know what a useful adjunct caffeine can be to food in mind and mood management, you may be wondering whether you *must* drink coffee, tea, or other caffeinated beverages in order to get the full benefits of these food/mind/mood strategies.

The answer, of course, is no. There are people who simply cannot tolerate caffeine even in low doses, much as they might want its obvious benefits. I have one client, for example, who has great difficulty organizing his thoughts in the morning. When he drinks coffee, he notices an immediate improvement in his ability to think on his feet, speak coherently and authoritatively, and respond quickly to questions. Thus, he always drank a cup of coffee before leaving home on days when he was scheduled to give morning sales presentations. But there was a problem. The increases in mental alacrity prompted by the caffeine was accompanied by distressing physical symptoms. Shortly after beginning a presentation, his hands would start to tremble, his palms would begin to sweat, and his stomach would become upset.

I suggested that he experiment and drink only half a cup of weak coffee before morning presentations. Unfortunately, even this smaller amount contained enough caffeine to cause physical discomfort. In the end, we decided it would be better for him to avoid all caffeine rather than continue to cut back in an effort to find the lowest possible dose that would benefit him without resulting in the side effects he feared. Obviously, if caffeine makes you as physically uncomfortable as it did my client, then you, too, should avoid it.

At the other end of the spectrum are people who drink coffee all day, almost as though it were water. Their caffeine tolerance is so high that they are immune to "coffee nerves." Although they usually experience the positive, brain-awakening effects that caffeine produces in others first thing in the morning, the jolt is not as pronounced, and successive cups do not seem to have the same valuable mind-mobilizing effect as with people who are more sensitive to the chemical. If you are a constant coffee drinker—for example, someone who can drink a cup or two at bedtime and then roll over and fall asleep—I'm afraid my caffeine strategy won't make much difference in your levels of mental energy. (But my food strategies will.)

My caffeine recommendations are for the large majority of

people who fall somewhere between these two extremes—
people who are able to tolerate two or three cups of coffee per
day without feeling jangled or suffering stomach upset, and yet
sensitive enough to caffeine to benefit from its mind- and
mood-managing properties.

If that sounds like you, coffee and other sources of caffeine
taken in moderation can be extremely valuable in helping you
achieve better mental energy and performance.

Common Major Sources of Caffeine

Coffee. A weak brew contains about 40 milligrams of
caffeine per cup, while strong espresso may have as
much as 200 milligrams per cup. Figure about 100
milligrams of caffeine per average cup.

Tea. Depending on type and length of brewing time, a cup
of tea contains between 40 and 80 milligrams of caffeine.

Cola-type soft drinks. Some brands contain as little as 30
milligrams of caffeine per twelve-ounce serving, others
as much as 60 milligrams.

Cocoa. Most commercial brands contain about 10 milligrams of caffeine per cup.

Assessing the Risk

As a scientist with a special interest in nutrition, an important part of my job is to keep up with the latest research
relating to my field. The studies done on caffeine are frequently contradictory. For every report indicating a link be-

tween caffeine and a major health problem, another, detailing research done by equally respected and disinterested investigators, indicates little or no such connection.

However, it has always seemed to me that if errors are to be made, they should be made on the side of caution.

My suggestion is that you consider the caffeine in coffee and other beverages as a chemical that, in view of all the evidence so far, is not harmful when consumed in relatively small amounts. But larger amounts are to be avoided.

I would define a relatively small amount of caffeine as between 200 and 300 milligrams a day, which is what you would get in two or three average cups of coffee.

These two or three cups, if you drink them according to the recommendations I have made in this chapter, are enough to give you two or three quick mental lifts, timed for when you need them most. But they are not enough, according to all the latest research, to present any hazards to your health. (I am not including stomach upsets and coffee nerves in the category of health hazards here, since they are both minor, temporary conditions, and easy to avoid simply by staying away from the culprit that caused them.)

However, if you are pregnant, think you might be, or are a nursing mother, please check with your doctor and follow his or her instructions regarding caffeine intake.

Caffeine and Fibrocystic Breast Disease

Perhaps the most alarming late-breaking news on caffeine as a health hazard are the reports that it is somehow linked to fibrocystic breast disease. However, there is so much confusion and misinformation about this connection that it merits some discussion.

Fibrocystic breast disease, loosely defined as a condition in which the breasts are lumpy and sore, is benign (noncancerous). But a certain type of benign lump is believed to be related to an increased risk of breast cancer.

Not all women whose breasts are occasionally lumpy and sore have fibrocystic breast disease. Not all breast lumps are fibrocysts, and not all women with benign breast lumps are candidates for developing malignant (cancerous) lumps.

A few years ago, a group of researchers claimed to have found a correlation between drinking coffee and other beverages containing caffeine and an increase in breast lumps and soreness. But the researchers did not make a distinction between different types of lumps. In the same report, it was claimed that when the women who participated in the study decreased their caffeine intake, there was a corresponding decrease in breast lumps and soreness.

One of the problems with this research was that everyone involved knew when the women were drinking high-caffeine beverages and when they had stopped. This raises the possibility of unconscious bias.

And even if there were fewer lumps when caffeine intake was reduced, we still do not know how many, if any, of the lumps that disappeared were the type that lead to cancer.

On the other hand, a report published in the April 1985 issue of the *Journal of the American Medical Association* compared the caffeine intake of two other groups of women. Some had lumpy, sore breasts; others were free of the condition. It was found that caffeine consumption of the two groups was identical. Moreover, the subjects in this study were unaware of any association between caffeine and breast lumps and were thus unlikely to be biased in reporting their actual coffee intake.

So we still do not know. Perhaps there is a connection between high caffeine intake, fibrocystic breast disease, and an increased risk of breast cancer. And perhaps not.

Given the contradictory nature of reports on the relation of caffeine to cancer and other diseases, one can only conclude that less is better than more, even though more may ultimately prove to be harmless.

Assuming that you *can* tolerate caffeine, limit your coffee intake to two or three cups a day, and time it so that each one delivers maximum brain power. You'll be staying well within limits virtually all respected researchers recognize as safe, while benefiting from the increased alertness and mental energy provided by this valuable mind and mood manager.

7. Meals That Really Work at Work

One of my most successful research collaborations—in fact, the one that ultimately led to my writing this book—got off the ground in a little coffee shop in Harvard Square. It was there that Dr. Bonnie Spring (then a member of the Harvard psychology department) and I met for lunch to work out the details of a study on how eating affects behavior.

The two of us were so enthusiastic, so engrossed in plotting an approach to our project, that we ran out of notebook paper and ended up scribbling on the napkins. I don't remember what we ate, but I think it must have been hamburgers because those napkins—precious because many of our key ideas were recorded on them—were spotted with ketchup.

Much of the work of the world is discussed, planned, negotiated at a table—over breakfast, lunch, or dinner. Not many business meals are as casual or productive as that one was for Dr. Spring and me. But as is the case with most working meals, the food was much less important than what we were attempting to accomplish.

Nevertheless, though filling your stomach may not be the primary purpose of a working meal, what you eat and how you eat it *can* influence your chances of success, whether you are trying to sell an idea, a product, a cause, or yourself as future employee or partner (or even as a son- or daughter-in-law).

Your choice of food can tip the scales in your favor by enhancing your mental alertness and your ability to communicate and respond with precision and authority. Or it can work against you by dulling your mind, slowing your reactions, and tying your tongue in knots.

What you eat at a business meal will also affect the way you perform and behave for an hour or so afterward, in that often all-important period when many of the details of a transaction are finalized.

I can't promise that if you order and eat according to my business meal guidelines, you always will leave the table with your objectives achieved. But I can guarantee that these few simple guidelines will help you perform up to your best potential. And, of course, when you are in top form the likelihood of getting what you want is increased!

The guidelines are basically the same for *any* working meal, whether it be an early morning strategy session, a lunchtime meeting for discussing a complex financial matter, or a getting-to-know-you dinner for people who will be working closely together in the future. The same five rules apply.

Rule 1.
Eat Sparingly

Not long ago I spent a few moments chatting with the maitre d' of a well-known Washington, D.C., restaurant where the power elite frequently meet for lunch or dinner. This voluble gentleman told me he could always tell who had the upper hand during a meal: "It's the one who orders mineral water, a clear soup, fish, and some vegetables, and then hardly touches his food. The guy who drinks, orders lavishly, and eats with gusto is going to be the loser in the deal," he said, nodding sagely.

He had arrived at his conclusions through day-in, day-out observation of the wheeling and dealing behaviors that are typically displayed at business meals. His conclusions coincide perfectly with mine, arrived at through laboratory testing and clinical work with patients and clients in my private practice.

Maximum mental performance during and after a working meal demands that you limit your calorie intake.

Do not eat more than about 400 calories at a working breakfast, and stay within the 500- to 600-calorie range at working lunches and dinners.

Obviously, I do not expect you to carry a calorie counter around with you so that you can slip it out of your pocket and calculate the exact number of calories supplied by so many ounces of this kind of meat or that kind of vegetable, etc. But I do suggest that in your spare time you do a bit of research on the caloric values of various foods so that you will know approximately how much you can eat and stay within these limits.

Here are just a few examples:

• *At breakfast,* a poached egg, a glass of juice, and a slice of very lightly buttered toast, plus coffee, would supply a little less than 400 calories. So would a bowl of unsweetened granola and low-fat milk—or low-fat yogurt with sliced fruit and a small muffin.

• *At lunch and dinner,* four to six ounces of fish, other seafood, or poultry with a vegetable or salad and clear soup are always good choices, adding up to between 500 and 600 calories.

But what if the portion sizes offered where your working meal takes place are gargantuan? Simple. Just don't eat everything on your plate.

Keeping the calorie content of a meal low always requires, in addition to limiting portion sizes, avoiding all fatty meats, fried foods, and most cheeses (the exceptions are cottage cheese, skim-milk ricotta, and mozzarella). Don't order anything served with a buttery or creamy sauce or blanketed in mayonnaise. If you order a salad, ask the waiter to serve dressing on the side, and use no more than three teaspoons. Dessert, if you have one, should be fresh fruit.

You may need to exercise some self-restraint, especially if you are being wined and dined at a restaurant known for its superb cuisine. But you cannot have your fill of rich, high-calorie food and expect to remain keen of mind and sharp of wit.

There is a direct relation between the number of calories consumed at a sitting and mental alertness. We've seen it demonstrated time and again in laboratory experiments: As calorie intake per meal is increased, mental performance afterward drops sharply.

You might even be slightly better off eating *fewer* calories than I have recommended!

This single recommendation—limit your calories at working meals—can lead to enormously gratifying results for you, as it has for some of my clients.

One of them, a lawyer who spends a great deal of time in Europe working out international patent agreements with foreign pharmaceutical firms, came to me because he thought he might be allergic to some of the ingredients in continental food. Negotiations with his European counterparts often took an entire day, but they were always interrupted by a long and lavish lunch. The meal usually included a first course of fish, followed by a richly sauced veal or chicken dish, potatoes and vegetables, and then salad. After the salad, cheese, bread, and crackers were served, and the meal finally ended with an extravagant dessert, often a butter cream–filled cake or ice cream and fruit sauce in a pastry shell.

My client said he felt sedated after these meals and that all his legal acumen vanished, only to be replaced by profound lethargy and a feeling of mental confusion.

I knew immediately that he wasn't suffering from an allergy, but from caloric overload, and told him next time to skip the meat, cheese, and dessert and just nibble at the fish, salad, and vegetables. "While you're at it, notice what the Europeans eat," I added.

When I saw him again, he told me that he had followed my suggestions and had just concluded a deal with terms very favorable to his firm.

But the really interesting thing, he said, was that the sharpest European negotiators at the table ate exactly as he did. "I watched one lawyer in particular, because he was the one I always had the most trouble with after lunch. He ate the fish, asked the waiter not to bring him any meat, toyed with the salad, refused the cheese, and ignored dessert. No wonder he was always wily as a fox after those lunches!"

Rule 2.
Don't Arrive Hungry

I had one client who dutifully followed my advice at a dinner meeting with some people who were looking him over as a possible consultant for their company. He ate half of the entrée, a small portion of rice, plain salad with no dressing, and ordered fruit for dessert.

Next time he came to my office I asked him how it went. "Fine, from the business end . . . I got the job. But," he went on, "I was so hungry that as soon as dinner was over I drove out to McDonald's for a Big Mac and some fries."

Why had he been so ravenous? His dinner had been small, but not *that* small. Well, he explained, he had not had time for lunch that day and in fact had eaten nothing since his breakfast bowl of cereal, early in the morning.

I'd forgotten to tell him Rule 2: *Never go to a business meal on an empty stomach.*

My client was able to overcome this handicap, I'm happy to say, but it could have been otherwise. In his famished state, all of his attention might have been focused on the food he wasn't supposed to eat rather than on making a positive presentation of himself, his ideas, and the contribution he could make to his potential clients.

Don't let what almost happened to this young man happen to you. If you haven't eaten for many hours, have a snack an hour before your business meal.

I usually advise clients to have some yogurt, a piece of fruit, a cup of clear soup, a bran muffin, or crackers and low-fat milk. The idea, of course, is *not* to fill up, but to eat just enough so that an hour or so later your mind won't be drawn to thoughts of food when you should be concentrating on the agenda of your working meal.

The exception to my snack-ahead rule is when your business meal is breakfast. Unless it is scheduled to begin several hours after you awaken, your hunger for this meal probably will not be so great that it interferes with your ability to concentrate on the conversation. However, if you wake up hungrier than usual, or if you exercise vigorously before your meeting, have a banana, a glass of milk, or a slice of toast as you dress.

If you are away from home and going to a business breakfast directly from your hotel, play it safe and bring something to snack on in the event that you feel hungry before the meeting. Single-serving boxes of cereal are ideal and travel well. Ring up room service for coffee or tea, and use some of the milk for your cereal.

You definitely *should* have a snack before a *late* business breakfast or brunch. A small bowl of cereal with low-fat milk, a muffin, or some cottage cheese and a slice of toast should be enough to hold you over.

If you are a coffee or tea drinker and a
your favorite beverage as soon as you
drink some before your morning meeting
early morning dose of caffeine, you r
inarticulate—and feeling and acting onl
the breakfast beverage arrives. This migl
few precious minutes of negotiating time. (If you travel with
an immersion heater, collapsible mug, and a small jar of
instant coffee or tea bags, as I do, you won't have to depend
on room service, which can be maddeningly slow when you
are in a rush.)

Timing is all. It is essential that you have your pre–business
meal snack about one hour before the meal itself. You want to
dull hunger so that you can zero in on your business objectives
instead of being distracted by a rumbling stomach and
thoughts of food. But you do not want to be so full that snack
plus meal add up to caloric overload and fuzzy-mindedness.

Rule 3.
Eat Protein Before Carbohydrate

This rule is extremely important for working lunches and
dinners, but somewhat less so for business breakfasts, which
occur early in the day, when the mind- and mood-modifying
properties of proteins and carbohydrates are barely
perceptible.

As for *why* you must ignore carbohydrates such as rolls,
bread, breadsticks, and other starchy or sweet foods at the
beginning of a business meal, the reason is simple: As you
know, when you start your meal with a carbohydrate, some of
the amino acid tryptophan will enter your brain and stimulate
it to make more serotonin, the calming chemical, and you will
begin to feel benign and relaxed.

Now, there is nothing wrong with feeling calm, benign, and
relaxed. It's the ideal state of mind to be in when you are off-

d taking your ease with family or friends. But it is not ur advantage to feel placid and agreeable when you are in usiness situation. You want your mental antennae quivering and alert. You want to be able to perceive and read accurately all the subtle nuances of proposal and counterproposal. You want your brain to be working at top speed so that you will be able to process information instantly and respond in ways that will advance your interests.

Avoiding carbohydrates at the beginning of a working meal will help you think better and stay mentally aroused and poised for action.

I have a client who was so interested in my advice about avoiding carbohydrates at the start of a business meal, that she decided to run a little experiment of her own. She wanted to see if she not only could enhance her own brain power with food but also give herself an additional negotiating edge by influencing what her customer, a buyer for a large computer outfit, ate as well.

She chose for dinner a restaurant that specialized in superb bread, made on the premises and served steaming hot in individual loaves with crocks of sweet butter. The bread *was* irresistible—although she, of course, ate none—and the service was slow enough so that her partner for the meal had time to consume an entire individual loaf before the waiter came to take their orders.

According to my client, she felt like a spider enticing a fly into a trap. The buyer was initially wary and determined not to make any concessions, but by the time the meal was half over, said my client, she could almost hear him purring. And she made sure they shook hands on the deal while he was still under the influence of all that serotonin!

Appetizers to Avoid

If you are going to follow my dictum of never starting a business meal with carbohydrates, make a mental note of these important food facts:

- All breads, crackers, rolls, chips, and appetizers made with rice, potatoes, pasta, or noodles are essentially carbohydrate. Avoid them.
- Any appetizer wrapped in fried dough, puff pastry, or baked in a pastry shell will, if the filling is vegetables or sauce rather than meat, be high enough in carbohydrates to start your brain producing serotonin. Ignore such appetizers.
- Bean and pea dishes such as bean soup, refried beans, baked beans, lentil soup, chickpea dip (hummus), nuts, and sunflower seeds are part protein, part carbohydrate. The protein component of these foods will block the amino acid tryptophan from achieving easy access to your brain and thus prevent a rush of serotonin production. However, foods in this category also tend to be filling and high in calories (nuts in particular are high in fat). So, in the interest of keeping your meal low in calories and avoiding brain drain, have these items only if you plan to order a *very* light main course. Otherwise, don't eat them.
- Pâté, though made with meat and thus a protein food, is also high in fat and calories. Pass it by.

Safe Meal Starters

As the list above indicates, many traditional appetizers and first courses are taboo. But there are still plenty of good, safe choices with which to begin a working meal:

- A clear soup such as consommé or chicken bouillon is virtually carbohydrate-free and low enough in calories not to cause an immediate overload. (But do not eat crackers or bread with your soup, and do *not* order creamed soup of any kind.)
- A simple green salad without croutons, served with a very light vinegar-and-oil dressing on the side, is fine.
- Shrimp cocktail, smoked salmon, smoked trout, pickled herring, oysters or clams on the half-shell (but not breaded

and baked), and other fish or seafood appetizers are excellent choices.

• Melon, grapefruit, and other fruits or fruit juices are good, too. Though they taste sweet and are indeed quite high in sugar, the sugar in fruit is fructose, which does not spur an immediate release of insulin from the pancreas. (As I explained earlier, an increase in insulin is the necessary first step in the complex process by which the brain is stimulated to make more serotonin.)

• Crunchy raw or marinated vegetables, provided the marinade is not too high in fat, are other excellent first course choices.

What should you do when your first course is your main course?

Easy. Give yourself a mental head start by beginning with the protein portion of your business meal. Eat slowly. By the time you have finished about half of your fish, lean meat, or poultry, there will be enough tyrosine in your system to sustain your brain's production of dopamine and norepinephrine, the alertness chemicals—and, just as important, to flood your body with amino acids that will block the manufacture of serotonin.

In watching people eat (a habit I can't or won't break), I have noticed that most men and women, when served a typical meal of fish, chicken, or beef accompanied by a potato or rice, will start with the carbohydrate, perhaps because it is easier to eat.

Lunching in a restaurant a few days ago, I noticed at a nearby table a man and woman obviously discussing business, since they kept referring to papers and charts in their respective briefcases. The man began with his steak and salad and left his potato for last. The woman, talking all the while, delayed eating until the waiter brought her some fresh-snipped chives to go with her baked potato. By the time the chives arrived, the man was halfway through his steak. Fascinated, I continued to watch. Her potato was a large one, and she didn't touch her own steak or salad until she had finished it—and all the while her brain was pumping out serotonin. I wondered as I paid my bill who eventually got the upper hand in their negotiations. But somehow I thought I knew.

Rule 4.
Order "Easy" Food

Now I'm going to suggest another guideline that has nothing to do with brain chemistry but will nevertheless help you concentrate on the agenda of your working meal:

I mentioned just a paragraph back that the temptation to eat carbohydrates first at a working meal may have to do with the fact that rice, potatoes, and other starches are so easy to eat. Nothing has to be cut, peeled, or speared, and all of one's attention can be given over to the business being transacted at the table.

Don't choose foods that require tricky manipulation with a knife, fork, or spoon; and above all, never try a new dish that you do not know how to eat. The reason is obvious: If you have to focus too hard on the physical act of eating, your attention will be sidetracked from the *real* business at hand.

Think before you order.

A few pointers:

- Broiled fish is always a good business meal choice, because it is low in calories and supplies the protein you need to stay in top mental form. But choose fish fillets, not a whole fish with bones that you will have to watch out for and remove as you eat.
- Boned chicken breasts require less knife-and-fork work than half a broiled chicken.
- Shrimp needs only to be cut into bite-sized pieces, but eating a whole lobster is a project in itself. If you crave lobster, have it in chunks or in a salad.

- Artichoke hearts are easier to eat than a whole artichoke. (And besides, it's next to impossible to maintain the pose of formidable adversary when you are pulling artichoke leaves through your teeth!)
- Rice and potatoes, of course, are simple. A small amount of either as part of your main course is preferable to long, slippery strands of spaghetti or linguine.
- Chinese, Japanese, and Korean specialties are often good choices, but don't use a working meal as a practice session for learning to eat with chopsticks. Unless you are already an expert, ask the waiter for Western-style utensils.

In short, stick with the easy, the tried and the true. Your working meals will be more productive.

Rule 5.
Avoid Alcohol

We've all heard of the hard-drinking businessman or woman who always clinches the deal, but how many of us have ever met one? That creature, I believe, is largely mythical.

It is certainly true that some people are more susceptible to the effects of alcohol than others, but no one is immune to this chemical. For some people—and you may be one of them—alcohol is initially stimulating. But the subsequent result of drinking more than a very small amount is always sedation.

A single drink before dinner or a glass of wine with your meal will begin to blunt your mind and weaken your powers of concentration at just about the time you are winding up your negotiations—even sooner if you arrived with an almost empty stomach.

The brain-dulling potential of alcohol is so great, so hazardous to the success of your working meal, that I do not even want to suggest a safe upper limit. There is none.

My advice with regard to alcohol is simple: *Order a drink*

before dinner only if not ordering one would call undue attention to yourself or inhibit your dining partners. When it arrives, take only a single sip and put the glass down. By drinking no more than a sip of alcohol you will be able to maintain your own mental alertness while that of the others at your table may be ebbing.

You will soon learn, as have many of my clients, that other people rarely notice whether you actually are drinking or not, as long as there is a glass of something in your hand or at your place. And that nearly full glass is a ready-made excuse when you are asked if you want a refill.

You can use the same tactic with wine during dinner. Allow your glass to be filled, take a single sip, and then switch to water. (Always ask your waiter to bring water; if there is none and you are very thirsty, you will surely be tempted to drink the wine.)

On those rare occasions when someone does notice that you are not really drinking, you can always say that you don't want the extra calories and then steer the conversation back to business. Believe me, the advantages of being clear-headed at the end of a meal—and beyond—are worth the occasional nuisance of having to explain to someone who is very proud of his or her wine expertise that you are trying to lose a pound or two. Indeed, I have noticed that such people are usually not adverse to taking my nearly full glass and finishing it off themselves!

Happy Endings

If the end of your meal is the end of your work for the day, then go ahead and treat yourself to a dessert if you like. Calorie overload at this point will be of no consequence in terms of managing your mind and your mood, since you will be winding down anyway. Even if you begin to feel slowed-down and fuzzy—as you will if dessert is a high-calorie concoction—it won't matter.

But if your meal will be followed by more work, further planning sessions or negotiations, or a report back to the boss, fruit is your best dessert choice. If fruit is unavailable? Then have nothing.

As for coffee or tea, take what you normally do. If you are accustomed to having a cup of either after lunch or dinner, eliminating it at a working meal is not a good idea. Habitual caffeine users tend to "crash" when levels of this chemical drop below a certain point. You don't want that to happen while you are still engaged in ironing out the details of a transaction or must continue working after your business meal.

If you do not usually drink a caffeinated beverage after meals, then there is no reason to end your business lunch or dinner with coffee or tea. Your system is not accustomed to it and doesn't require it. Have herb tea or decaffeinated coffee instead.

These strategies for working meals that *really* work may seem stringent, and you will need to exercise self-control to follow them. Most of all, they require that you think about working meals less as pleasurable opportunities to fill up on food and drink and more as opportunities to contribute, achieve, and advance professionally or socially. Once you have made this shift in viewpoint, the battle is mostly won. The food you choose—what you eat and how and when you eat it—will do the rest.

Try it, and you'll see exactly what I mean.

8. Preperformance Meals: Eating for a Winning Presentation

We all have to perform from the moment we arise in the morning to the time we finally close our eyes at night. But that's not the kind of performing I'm concerned with in this chapter.

Rather, I'm going to tell you how to eat for those special occasions when you are putting yourself on the line—giving a speech or making a presentation, taking an exam, interviewing for a job, auditioning for a television spot. As in so many other situations, the state of your brain, and the chemicals it is producing as a result of what you do or don't eat beforehand, can make a vital difference.

You, of course, will have to learn your speech, memorize the figures for your presentation, cram for your test, prepare for your interview, or practice your lines until you can say them in your sleep. But these preperformance meal strategies will help ensure that you will be alert, not tense and edgy, that you will be focused, not mentally immobilized, that you will think quickly and accurately, without being hyper.

You will notice that some of these guidelines for preperformance eating are similar to the working meal suggestions made in the previous chapter. This is because the principles of eating to achieve and maintain optimum brain power are basically the same for all demanding situations.

However, in the last chapter, we were concerned with how to eat *during* important business or social transactions. Here we're going to explore the idea of using food to prime your mind *beforehand,* to rev up your mental machinery in advance so that you will be fully prepped to meet any upcoming challenge with increased potential for success.

Here is a rundown of the basic principles that apply particularly to preperformance eating:

1. Choose food low in calories and fat.
2. Drink enough coffee or tea ahead of time to maintain your body's usual level of caffeine throughout your performance. (This rule, obviously, applies to coffee and tea drinkers only. If you rarely drink either, you should *not* attempt to use caffeine to increase mental alertness before a performance. Your system isn't used to it, and pouring in unaccustomed amounts of caffeine may increase your nervousness.)
3. Drink little or no alcohol on the day of your performance; drink *no* alcohol in the three hours prior to your presentation.
4. If possible, time preperformance eating so that it occurs about two hours before you must go on.
5. Never perform on a completely empty stomach.

Timing
Your Preperformance Meal

Digestion is a complex process that begins when food is chewed and swallowed and may take several hours to complete. As I have mentioned elsewhere, the heavier the meal and the more fat it contains, the longer digestion will take. While your food is moving slowly through the various stages of digestion, relatively more blood flows to the stomach and other organs involved in the process, making less blood available to your brain.

Now, with regard to blood supply, you want your brain to take precedence over your digestive tract during a performance. When it doesn't, the result is diminished alertness, a measurable decrease in cerebral activity, and slowed-down responses.

An empty stomach, however, can be just as detrimental as an overly full stomach that is actively engaged with digestion. Going for several hours without food may make you feel weak and queasy, even give you a headache.

Besides that, hunger is distracting and interferes with concentration.

The way to avoid both performance handicaps—the mental fogginess that accompanies calorie overload and the distractibility and weakness associated with hunger—is to eat a small meal consisting of light, low-fat food about two hours before you must meet your mental challenge.

If you have one of the simple low-fat, low-carbohydrate meals I am going to recommend in this chapter, within the two-hour safety eating zone, the part of digestion in which blood is diverted away from your brain and to your gut will be completed by the time you perform, but hunger still will be a long way off.

How to Prime Your Mind for a Morning Performance

A good preperformance breakfast must be substantial enough to satisfy hunger after your seven- or eight-hour overnight fast, yet light enough and low enough in fat for quick, easy digestion.

One of my clients, a grants administrator at a large university who also runs competitively, told me that the morning preperformance menus I gave her were similar to the breakfasts her running coach suggested for race days. I wasn't surprised to hear it. There *are* parallels between the vigorous mental effort required to excel in a speech or presentation and the physical demands of competing in an athletic event. Both depend on careful preparation for success. Both trigger the stress-related mechanism that pumps adrenaline into the bloodstream and sets the heart to beating faster in anticipation of meeting a challenge. *And* it's almost impossible to win in either situation if you are handicapped by poor preperformance eating—by having too much mind- and body-slowing food bogged down in the intestinal tract, on the one hand, or by a debilitating insufficiency of calories and other nutrients, on the other.

The following three light, low-fat breakfasts have helped many of my clients meet and master the mental demands of a morning speech, test, or other performance scheduled for early in the day. Did these breakfasts actually *improve* their mental capabilities? The only way to know for sure would be to have these people repeat their performances under the exact same circumstances but after eating different breakfasts. Obviously, that kind of testing is not possible.

I do know, however, that these clients all were convinced that they achieved their full performance potential after eating the breakfasts we prescribed. I think you will be, too.

PREPERFORMANCE BREAKFAST #1
½ grapefruit or 4 ounces orange or other fruit juice
1 poached egg
1 slice whole-grain toast, dry or very lightly buttered
Coffee or tea as usual

PREPERFORMANCE BREAKFAST #2
½ grapefruit or 4 ounces orange or other fruit juice

½ cup oatmeal with
½ cup low-fat or skim milk
Coffee or tea as usual

PREPERFORMANCE BREAKFAST #3
1 medium sliced peach, apple, or banana, or ½ cup sliced berries
    mixed into
¾ cup cottage cheese or plain low-fat yogurt
1 small corn or bran muffin, dry or very lightly buttered
Coffee or tea as usual

When to Eat

It's worth getting up early in order to get one of these breakfasts into your system within the safety eating period of about two hours before your performance.

The A.M. Coffee Factor

You will notice that in each of the menus above, I have included the directive "coffee or tea as usual." Although the effects of caffeine are long-lasting and diminish very gradually over a number of hours, the level of caffeine in your system after a full night's sleep will be close to zero. So if you can tolerate it, a cup of coffee or tea can be an extremely valuable tool for priming the brain for mental effort and even improving powers of articulation.

Even if you know that coffee or tea will be served at your meeting, interview, or test center, do not wait until you get there to have your first morning caffeine. It may be too late. Better to arrive already mentally primed.

Food Tactics for an Early-Morning Performance

Let's say that you are scheduled to speak or give a presentation as part of a breakfast meeting and that food will be served just prior to the start of the program. Should you sit down with your colleagues and coworkers and have an additional bite to eat with them, just to be sociable? The answer, of course, is no—not if you want to perform at your peak.

Eat before you leave your home or hotel. Then avoid all other food until after your performance. If you want to join your colleagues at the breakfast table beforehand, sip coffee or tea only—decaffeinated, if more than one cup of a caffeinated beverage in the morning makes you feel jangled.

In particular, be wary of the sweet rolls, croissants, doughnuts, and other high-calorie, high-fat goodies that often are set out at morning meetings. Eating even one of them will defeat the purpose of your light, low-fat breakfast by contributing to preperformance digestive overload and the slowed-down mental state that always goes with it.

I had a client who often was required to give four-hour lectures to large groups of graduate students. Her talks typically began at eight in the morning and ran until noon. She came to me because always within minutes of beginning to speak she felt "blurry," as she put it, and became less articulate.

In response to my question about what she ate before her talks, she told me that she usually left home at seven with an empty stomach but filled up on a cheese omelet, bacon, hashbrowned potatoes, and toast at a coffee shop just before entering the lecture hall. I explained the principles of light, low-fat eating and why meals should be taken at least an hour before she had to perform. I also remarked on the importance of mind-priming caffeine. (She is a moderate coffee drinker.) She agreed to follow my suggestions in preparing for her next talk.

When I saw her again and asked if my preperformance breakfast tactics had helped, her answer was, "Not really." In fact, she said, she felt as blurred as ever when she ate according to my recommendations.

Her experience ran counter to everything we know about

the food/mind/mood response, and I began to wonder if she might have an undiagnosed physical problem. But no. As we continued our discussion, she mentioned stopping off at the coffee shop for a cheese Danish just before her lecture. It was this last-minute pastry, high in calories and fat, eaten on top of breakfast, that prevented her from obtaining the benefits of the peak performance food guidelines!

On the morning of her next lecture she followed the guidelines to the letter and skipped the Danish. This time she was able to breeze through her grueling four-hour talk, remaining clear-headed and not bothered by the inarticulate pauses that had hampered her performances in the past.

Food Tactics for a Late-Morning Performance

What if your speech or interview is set for later in the morning, say, after the coffee break, which is usually scheduled for ten-thirty or so?

The basic tactics remain the same: Before you leave home or your hotel, eat one of the light, low-fat breakfasts listed in chapter 5. Drink a cup of coffee or tea along with it if you usually have a caffeinated beverage in the morning.

Then, at coffee break, socialize if you like, or find a quiet spot to study your speech or run through your presentation one last time (unless you are a carbohydrate craver—if you are, see the Carb Cravers' Alert, coming up).

If you had breakfast at eight or even seven, your system still will be supplied with enough calories at eleven or so to prevent real hunger. ("Fake hunger" is another matter. If you ordinarily have a snack at midmorning, your stomach may be accustomed to something to eat at about this time. Be prepared to exercise some self-control.)

You *must* stay away from the high-calorie, high-fat, high-carbohydrate croissants, sweet rolls, and doughnuts that are coffee break staples. Eating a heavy starch now, only minutes before you must perform, will slow you down, dull your mental processes, and possibly result in some loss of verbal facility.

Carb Craver's Alert!

If you feel very jittery or tense midmorning, and the food/mind/mood demonstration test in chapter 4 indicated that you are a carbohydrate craver, your high anxiety level may be the result of a fall-off in brain serotonin. A very light, low-fat restorative snack consisting of one or one and a half ounces of sweet or starchy food (such as a muffin, rice cakes, saltines, or an ounce of jelly beans) will trigger the production of more serotonin, which will in turn calm you and help you to focus your mind. For what to eat, see the carbohydrate snacks listed in Appendix A.

The Coffee Break Caffeine Question

You already know my stand on wake-up coffee or tea: If you usually have a caffeinated beverage on arising, it is important not to deviate from routine on mornings when you must perform.

But the decision to have a second cup at coffee break, just before you are scheduled to speak, be interviewed, or take an oral or written test, must be based on your sensitivity to this chemical.

The brain-sharpening effects of caffeine linger on for several hours after you drink a cup of coffee or tea. If you had some at breakfast—and if your sensitivity to caffeine is about average—you won't need another caffeine pickup for several hours. In fact, more caffeine just now might make you too hyper to perform at your potential.

If you consider yourself average in terms of caffeine sensitivity, *don't* have more regular coffee or tea during the break. There are several less risky alternatives:

- Decaffeinated coffee or tea
- Herb tea
- Fruit juice

- Seltzer or mineral water
- Plain ice water

FOR CAFFEINE ADDICTS ONLY. The no-caffeine-at-coffee-break rule above does *not* apply to you if you regularly drink eight, ten, or twelve cups of coffee or tea daily and your caffeine tolerance is so high that you are immune to the nerve-jangling effect it can have on others. In fact, for you, a sharp drop in the amount of caffeine in your system can be just as detrimental to delivering a top-notch performance as too much caffeine would be to someone more sensitive to the chemical.

If you drink gallons of coffee or tea each day, I suggest you seriously consider cutting back. But until you do, it is important, when you are in a mentally demanding situation, to keep caffeine levels up to what is normal for you.

How to Eat for a Top Afternoon Performance

When you are scheduled to speak, be interviewed, tested, or auditioned in the afternoon, the meal you should be most concerned with, of course, is lunch.

The ideal lunch for enhancing peak performance potential, like the ideal preperformance breakfast, is very light and low in fat, and for the same reasons: to maximize mental alertness and brain power and prevent the slowed responses and loss of verbal facility that result from calorie overload.

However, before we go on to the dos and don'ts of eating for an afternoon performance, let's backtrack a moment.

Major Breakfast, Minor Lunch: The Crucial Keys to P.M. "Star Quality"

Because lunch *must* be small, it is important not to skimp on breakfast.

Unfortunately, I learned this the hard way, as did one of my clients. In counseling her to keep lunch as small and as low in fat and carbohydrates as possible, I did not at first take into consideration the fact that unless she ate a substantial breakfast, she might be too famished to adhere to my luncheon guidelines or too hungry after a very light lunch to perform at peak.

A musician, this client told me that by the time she was called on to play, she had a headache and was slightly queasy, a condition she attributed to sheer nerves. But when I questioned her about breakfast, she told me that she never ate it, which convinced me that her preaudition queasiness was caused as much by hunger as by nerves.

Now, when a client must be at his or her mental sharpest in the afternoon, I always advise starting the day with a breakfast substantial enough to prevent hunger from interfering with my light lunch recommendations or with the performance that follows.

On days when you must face a tough mental challenge in the afternoon, start out in the morning with one of the following "major" breakfasts.

MAJOR BREAKFAST #1
½ grapefruit or 4 ounces fruit juice
2 eggs, poached or soft-boiled
1 slice Canadian bacon (which is leaner than the ordinary kind)
1 bagel with pat of butter
Coffee or tea as usual

MAJOR BREAKFAST #2
½ grapefruit or 4 ounces fruit juice
1 cup oatmeal mixed with
¼ cup raisins and ½ sliced banana
Bran or corn muffin with pat of butter
Coffee or tea as usual

MAJOR BREAKFAST #3
½ grapefruit or 4 ounces fruit juice
1 cup cottage cheese or plain yogurt mixed with

½ cup sliced fruit, such as apple, peach, berries, and
½ cup granola
2 slices toast with pat of butter
Coffee or tea as usual

Ordering Your Own Preperformance Lunch

Now that you know why you must have a substantial breakfast on days when you must perform well in the afternoon, let's consider the meal that will most directly influence your afternoon brain power: lunch.

As I explained earlier, it should be light and low in calories, fat, and carbohydrate. You will have the greatest degree of control over these variables if you pack your own lunch or go out to a nearby non-specialty restaurant where you can be sure of getting the kind of food that will best enhance your upcoming performance. Any of the following three menus will do just that:

PREPERFORMANCE LUNCH MENU #1
3 ounces very lean roast beef on
1 slice whole-grain bread
1 apple
Coffee or tea as usual

PREPERFORMANCE LUNCH MENU #2
Chef's salad made with 1½ cups salad greens, *no dressing*, and 1 ounce feta cheese, 1 ounce white meat chicken, 1 ounce lean roast beef
1 small whole-grain roll, no butter
Coffee or tea as usual

PREPERFORMANCE LUNCH MENU #3
3 ounces broiled nonoily fish such as haddock, halibut, sole, or flounder, or 3 ounces water-packed tuna
½ cup rice or ½ baked potato, with *no* butter or sour cream
½ cup fresh fruit cocktail, made *without* sugar
Coffee or tea as usual

Catered Preperformance Lunches

Unfortunately, you won't always be able to make or order your own preperformance lunch. Instead you will have to make do with food selected by a caterer, conference planning committee, or even the boss's secretary.

But you can always control how much you eat and keep your calorie, fat, and carbohydrate consumption down to safe levels if you follow these recommendations:

- Eat no more than three ounces of chicken, meat, or fish. Remove chicken skin or carefully trim all visible fat from meat. Scrape away any rich gravy or sauce. (You'll want to do this as inconspicuously as possible, of course.)
- Have a small serving of vegetables—one-half cup or less. (High-fiber vegetables such as broccoli, cabbage, and brussels sprouts are low in calories, but they may slow digestion and make you feel uncomfortably bloated.) If vegetables are served with a fatty sauce—Hollandaise, for example—ask the waiter to bring yours unadorned. Other options: Scrape off the sauce or simply skip the vegetables. You can do without them for this one meal.
- If a salad is served, ask for dressing on the side and use it *very* sparingly. If salad comes to the table already covered with a thick creamy or oily dressing, don't eat it.
- Limit your starch intake to one-half cup of rice or half a baked potato (no butter or sour cream) or a small roll or slice of bread, unbuttered.
- A cup of clear soup or consommé is fine, but pass on creamy or fatty soups.
- Avoid hard cheeses, fried foods of any kind, gravy, and mayonnaise. All are too high in fat for a preperformance lunch.
- If the entrée is heavy and highly calorific—fettucini Alfredo, for example, or moussaka or seafood Newburg—take just a bite or two, and concentrate instead on the

appetizer (if it is low in fat), salad, vegetables, and soup (if it is a plain consommé or clear soup). I call this tactic "eating around the entrée," and it has been extremely useful to many of my clients.

- Have unsweetened fresh or stewed fruit for dessert, if it is available. All other desserts are taboo.
- End your meal with a cup of coffee or tea if you usually have a caffeinated beverage after lunch.

The idea, obviously, is to eat less than you normally do. In fact, the lighter and lower in calories, fat, and carbohydrates your lunch is, the better it will serve your preperformance needs.

Ideally, you should leave the table feeling not quite satisfied. I am *not* suggesting that you go entirely without eating, however. Fasting isn't necessary and won't improve your mental capabilities. But a light lunch consisting of three ounces of protein and one-half cup of a carbohydrate food will!

The Nervous-Eating Syndrome and How to Beat It

For many people the act of eating is a tension-reliever. Some of my clients tell me that they know they have, on a subconscious level, attempted to deal with preperformance stage fright by filling up on food.

I remember one client in particular who *hated* to speak in front of an audience but whose job required that he do so at least once a month. In his own words, he "sweated bullets" before these talks, which usually were scheduled as part of a luncheon meeting. At these preperformance lunches, he said, his mind would be fixed on the upcoming ordeal, while his body functioned almost like a motor-driven robot, fork moving from plate to mouth and back again, shoveling in the food until every last morsel was consumed.

He told me that he always felt awful after overeating—"as though my stomach were loaded with lead, and my head stuffed with wool." However, he thought these distressing symptoms were manifestations of his fear of public speaking.

When I explained that calorie overload was actually the *cause* of much of his mental and physical preperformance stress, he agreed to follow my suggestions and eat a very light, low-calorie lunch before his next talk.

I'm pleased to say he was amazed at how much better he felt and performed when he ate fewer calories and less fat and carbohydrates before speaking. He still feels somewhat nervous before a talk, and he is still tempted on occasion to use food to ease his anxiety. But because he does not want to miss out on the proven benefits of a light preperformance meal, he devised his own insurance policy to prevent calorie overload: At luncheon meetings, he eats about three ounces of the protein he is served, and one-half cup (or its equivalent) of the carbohydrate. Then he stands up, excuses himself, and leaves the table, ostensibly for the men's room. He stays away until his plate is removed, and with it the possibility that he might overeat.

I've recommended this trick to several clients, and it always seems to work. Try it.

Food Tactics to Boost a Late-Afternoon Performance

When you are scheduled to perform late in the afternoon, you don't need to be concerned about breakfast or restrict your calories quite so much at lunch. Assuming you don't overeat, by four o'clock your lunch will be in your system long enough so that large amounts of blood no longer need to be diverted to your digestive tract.

But there are still a couple of steps you can take to maximize late afternoon performance potential. One is a do, and the other is a don't.

• *Do have a cup of coffee, tea, or a soft drink containing caffeine about an hour before you make your presentation.*

This recommendation applies to just about everyone. Caffeine in the afternoon, when your body and mind are beginning to wind down for the day, will enhance alertness, mental energy, and verbal facility. If you are a light to moderate coffee or tea drinker, you certainly will want another cup just about now in order to maintain the usual high level of caffeine in your system.

The only people who should *not* take caffeine an hour before a late-afternoon performance are those who are so supersensitive to this chemical that it leaves them feeling shaky and on edge for hours after it is ingested.

• *Don't eat a carbohydrate snack until after your performance.*

Carbohydrate is the right thing to eat in many afternoon situations, but not this one. When you must give a speech or otherwise present yourself professionally to best advantage, you want to be quick-witted and vibrating with energy, your brain keyed up, not toned down.

You would think that I, of all people, would not make the mistake of eating a carbohydrate food before an afternoon performance. But I forgot to take my own advice once and ate a corn muffin before a five o'clock afternoon television interview.

At four-forty-five I strolled into the studio, wondering why I felt so relaxed. Half an hour or so later, with the cameras rolling and the television talk show host firing questions at me, I realized I was altogether *too* relaxed. My ability to frame short, concise, appropriate, and witty answers to his machine-gun questions was nil. Needless to say, it was not one of my best performances.

Later on, trying to figure out why I had meandered so during this particular interview, I remembered the corn muffin. What a difference even a small amount of the wrong food at the wrong time can make!

If you are truly hungry and need something to eat before a late-afternoon performance, have a "neutral" food (one that will have no impact on your mood and behavior) such as an apple or other fruit. Better still, have a few ounces of protein in the form of one-half cup cottage cheese or plain yogurt, or a hard-boiled egg. They'll rev up your mind instead of slowing it down.

Carb Cravers' Alert!

If you frequently feel distracted, unfocused, edgy, or irritable late in the afternoon, you are the exception to the above. Unlike most people, you *should* have a light, low-fat carbohydrate snack shortly before an afternoon performance. One to one and one-half ounces of a sweet or starchy food will stimulate serotonin production in your brain, quickly restoring your ability to focus your thoughts, and moderating your mood. Choose from the list of carbohydrate snacks given in Appendix A.

Eating to Star at an Evening Performance

It has always seemed to me that speaking after dinner is a chore (especially after a long, hard day at work). It is usually a bore as well, for speechifier and listeners alike. Nevertheless there comes a time in almost every professional man or woman's life when the obligation to say a few words at a dinner meeting is unavoidable.

Your main objective as after-dinner speaker is to be at least as awake and alert as your audience—if possible, to inform, inspire, and/or entertain. I can't help you put together a scintillating speech, but I can give you guidelines that will help you stay wide awake, mentally energetic, and articulate throughout your ordeal. You've heard them before: Eat very sparingly beforehand, get protein into your system before carbohydrate, and avoid alcohol.

Now for the specifics.

When possible, eat at home before your after-dinner performance.

This piece of advice always seems to surprise my clients. After all, why miss out on a free and probably sumptuous meal? Why indeed? Because it is always easier to control the amount and kind of food you eat—and thus help yourself to better performance potential—when you cook it yourself.

I was delighted to learn a few years ago that not every after-dinner speech carries with it the obligation to dine with your audience. I made this discovery when I was delayed at a late afternoon meeting and called the M.C. of the dinner meeting I would be addressing later to tell him I would have to miss the meal but would be there in time for my talk. "No problem," he assured me. And ever since, when accepting a speaking engagement, I often say I can't be there for the dinner but will arrive in time for dessert (which I do not eat), coffee, and, of course, my talk.

Frankly, my reluctance to eat *and* speak at a dinner meeting has almost as much to do with needing a break in my working day as with controlling my food intake and ensuring a good performance. Instead of sitting at a banquet table for ninety minutes, nibbling very selectively at the food, I'd rather spend the time at home, where I can exercise, have a small, low-calorie meal of my own choosing, and then relax for a while before going out to speak.

The following menus, all light and low in fats and carbohydrates, are excellent choices for at-home dining before an after-dinner speech.

AT-HOME PREPERFORMANCE DINNER #1

4–5 ounces chicken breast (skinned) poached in broth

1 cup of stir-fried vegetables (broccoli, snow peas, carrots, mushrooms)

½ cup white or brown rice
¾ cup fresh strawberries or ½ grapefruit
1 cup skim milk (optional)

AT-HOME PREPERFORMANCE DINNER #2
5 ounces baked fish or scallops with ginger*
½ cup of Chinese noodles
½–¾ cup steamed broccoli
Fresh pear or apple
1 cup skim milk (optional)

AT-HOME PREPERFORMANCE DINNER #3
2-egg mushroom omelet cooked with no more than 1 teaspoon
    butter or margarine
1 English muffin with ¼ cup skim milk ricotta cheese
Baked apple (optional)

Dinner Meeting Eating Tactics

To be realistic, however, you will not always be able to skip the dinner portion of an evening speaking engagement. The question then becomes, how do you negotiate your way through the appetizers and soup, the salad and entrée, and finally the dessert without succumbing to mind-numbing calorie overload and possibly turning in a poor performance?

The two-part answer is: Have a snack three or four hours before you are scheduled to speak so that hunger won't get the better of you at dinner. Then eat as lightly as possible when the meeting meal is served.

As I mentioned in the lunch section of this chapter, without a snack a few hours beforehand, you may be too ravenous to follow my light-eating guidelines—or too hungry after your very low-calorie dinner to speak with the ease, verve, and conviction that mark a memorable talk.

*See recipe in Appendix B.

Select from the three predinner snack alternatives below. Each supplies enough calories to subdue hunger but is light enough to be quickly and easily digested.

PREDINNER SNACK #1
1 cup vegetable soup
2–3 ounces chicken or lean beef on
1 slice whole-grain bread with *no* butter or mayonnaise

PREDINNER SNACK #2
1 cup plain, coffee-, lemon-, or vanilla-flavored yogurt
1 bran or corn muffin, unbuttered

PREDINNER SNACK #3
1–2 ounces cheese (any kind, but avoid salty cheeses, as these may make you thirsty during your presentation)
1 medium apple
3 wheat or rye crackers, unbuttered

BRAIN-POWERING GUIDELINES FOR BANQUET EATING. All of the preperformance lunch tactics for catered meals just discussed will help prevent the lethargy and slowed responses resulting from digestive overload. Go back and take a look at them. Team them with the suggestions below to maintain mental alertness and further enhance your eating performance potential:

- Don't eat carbohydrates before you eat protein. It is now late in the day and your mind and body are in a winding-down mode—*drowsy.* As you know, eating carbohydrate before protein in the evening is almost like taking a sleeping pill. Conversely, eating protein before carbohydrate will block the manufacture of serotonin and keep you keen-minded and prepared to perform at peak.
- Say "No, thank you" when the hors d'oeuvres are passed. Exceptions are plain boiled or broiled shrimp and other seafood and crunchy raw vegetables. These are all

safe, in that they are very low in calories and carbohydrates. (Vegetables, however, should be eaten plain, not dunked in a creamy or oily dip.) Eat very little even of these relatively harmless hors d'oeuvres, since like *all* food, they take up space in your stomach and contribute to digestive overload.

- Finish about one-third of each dish that is part of the main course. (Remember, begin with protein—meat, fish, other seafood, or poultry. Do not eat any rice, potato, or other starchy food until you have finished one-third of the protein on your plate. If the starchy component of your meal is fried or comes to the table lavished with butter or a creamy or cheesy sauce, don't eat it at all.)

- Have coffee or tea at the end of your meal if your caffeine tolerance is about average and you usually have a caffeinated beverage at about this time, or if it has been several hours since your last cup. Caffeine on top of a low-calorie meal that begins with protein will quicken your responses and stimulate cerebral activity, putting you in top form when you finally go on.

  Important note to the nervous: Though caffeine at the end of a preperformance dinner is usually a help, it can be a hindrance if speaking in front of a group makes you feel overwhelmed with anxiety. When that is the case, make it a point to have coffee or tea an hour or so *before* dinner, so that the caffeine levels in your system will be somewhat diminished by the time you speak. A fresh injection of caffeine when you are quivering with preperformance nerves may make you feel too agitated and too shaky to deliver a smooth, coherent presentation.

THE MAN WHO KNEW BUT DIDN'T DO. It is not enough to understand the food tactics for achieving a star-quality performance. Reading about food won't make it work for you. Knowing what to do isn't good enough by itself. You must follow through.

A client of mine, for example, a brilliant political scientist, could recite my food guidelines back to me verbatim. He knew exactly how to eat to enhance a performance. But when he was invited to speak to a society known for the excellence of its food and wine, he chose to disregard what he had learned and decided instead to savor the meal.

Since my client was watching his weight at the time, he thought it would be a good idea to save a few calories by skipping lunch and not snacking in the afternoon before his speech. Predictably, he was hungry when he arrived at the meeting. Just as predictably, he was mentally ready for bed by the time he had eaten a dozen small batter-dipped hors d'oeuvres before dinner; worked his way through the appetizer—a creamy salmon mousse; consumed a half-pound serving of roast beef accompanied by sautéed potatoes and butter-drenched string beans amandine and, finally, polished off an elegant hazel nut torte (not to mention drinking a different wine with each course).

He told me later that his brain "felt like a car engine that wouldn't turn over on a cold morning." The audience expected wit, intelligence, and insight, he said, "and what they got was stumbling and bumbling. It was an embarrassment."

"Coming Down" for a Good Night's Sleep

The party's over, your performance was a success, and now you are on a mental high. At this point in the evening, after keeping your appetite in check for so long, you may be hungry or at least feel you deserve something to eat. You do. But the food choices you make now are important, too.

Eat protein and your brain may begin to make more of the alertness chemicals, dopamine and norepinephrine—the last thing you need, since you are probably already mentally stimulated more than is normal for you this late in the day. In fact, a protein snack could keep you tossing and turning for hours, reliving over and over again in your mind the excitement of the evening.

Instead, assuming that the hour is late, you should eat something that will slow your thoughts, something that will help you relax, begin to feel drowsy, and fall asleep soon after you crawl into bed. Carbohydrate, of course, will do all of this.

As little as one to one and one-half ounces of a carbohydrate food—starch or sweet—will do it if your weight is about where it should be. If you are seriously overweight, you may have to eat an additional ounce or two to obtain its calming benefits.

Any carbohydrate food will induce your brain to make more serotonin, but I have discovered that the following are especially valuable postperformance relaxers:

- Three or four cookies, such as plain vanilla wafers, ginger snaps, sugar wafers, fig bars, or cookies filled with marshmallow or jam
- A granola bar
- A toaster corn or bran muffin
- Two toaster waffles or frozen French toast with two teaspoons maple syrup
- A single plain or sugar doughnut
- One cup low-fat ice cream
- A cup of cocoa made with real sugar (i.e., not dietetic) and topped with one tablespoon marshmallow fluff
- One to one and a half cups instant hot cereal with one tablespoon honey or brown sugar
- A small package of candy such as gumdrops, licorice bits, jelly beans, or part-chocolate candies such as M&M's or a Snickers or Zero bar. (Pure chocolate is too high in fat for quick digestion and thus takes longer to stimulate production of relaxing serotonin.)

I never tell my clients—and I won't tell you—that eating to increase performance potential is easy. You may have to set your alarm to go off an hour or so early or otherwise reshuffle your schedule in order to prime your mind by getting the right food into your system at the right time. You probably will have to eat less of some of the things you like best and may have to turn down some of your favorite dishes at a preperformance lunch or dinner. But clients who have followed my suggestions agree that these small sacrifices are nothing compared to the satisfaction of knowing they have achieved their very best performance capabilities.

One client, a university professor, followed these guidelines before speaking at a black-tie dinner. He summed up his experience of that evening rather nicely: "I don't know if the food I ate made me the hit of the meeting, but it was the best presentation I ever gave, and that made me a hit with myself."

9. Conference-Goers' Guide to High-Achievement Eating

I'd like to tell you about a client, a young Navy officer who was doing postgraduate work at M.I.T. During his year in Cambridge, Massachusetts, Uncle Sam requested his presence at a number of two- and three-day meetings in Annapolis and Washington.

"It's peculiar how I always go to these workshops feeling terrific," he said. "I'm full of energy, motivated, eager to learn the latest techniques in my field. Yet by day two, I'm having trouble concentrating, feeling lethargic, and can't seem to follow the gist of things. What puzzles me most is that I *know* the material covered at the workshops is easier than most of the stuff I have to master at M.I.T. But it *seems* more difficult!"

His story had a familiar ring. It wasn't the first time I had encountered someone whose brain turned to mush at an all-day or longer conference. In fact, I see the phenomenon so often I've given it a name: the Conference Blahs.

The Conference Blahs—
Causes and Cures

Why do so many conference-goers experience a sharp decline in mental alertness and acuity within hours after they arrive on the premises? Why do so many of them feel as though they are sleepwalking through the proceedings? And why do they so often miss out on the unique and valuable opportunities a conference offers—opportunities to contribute, to learn, to expand their range of business contacts, and to score important professional points, thereby advancing their own and their firms' interests?

It's very simple. At the typical conference, attendees are fed two, if not three, high-calorie, high-fat, high-carbohydrate meals each day, and built into the schedule will be one or two coffee breaks offering more of the same *wrong* foods. Add to that the fact that most of the time will be spent sitting (except for those in charge of a booth or display, who will spend their days standing), with little opportunity for exercise, and it becomes obvious: Unless the conference-goer knows how to eat for maximum mental energy and productivity, attention will lag, performance will sag, chances to advance will be lost. An expanded waistline will be the most notable gain from the experience.

A forty-year-old woman who has exhibited for the last five years at gift shows across the country came to me because by the end of each season she had gained twenty-five to thirty pounds. "It gets so boring answering the same questions about sizes and prices over and over again," she said. "And it's so tedious standing in that little booth. I can hardly wait for the food breaks. In fact, I pass the time thinking about what I'm going to eat next."

Was she at least pleased with her sales records at these shows, I asked. "No," was the reply. "I'm sure I could do better if I didn't feel so sluggish and fatigued all the time."

It needn't be that way for you. It shouldn't be. Whether you go to several conferences a year or only occasionally, you owe it to yourself to function at peak efficiency, to maintain a focused, alert mind the whole time so that you can assimilate each new piece of information that comes your way, grasp every new technique, cultivate every new contact. Otherwise, why bother to attend?

The food/mind/mood tactics that will keep you in top mental form from the moment you arrive at conference headquarters should be familiar to you by now. They are essentially the same as my guidelines for maintaining a competitive edge during a business meeting and for priming your mind for a successful speech, interview, test, or audition. This time around I'm going to tell you how to use them to take full advantage of a conference situation.

First, for ready reference, here's a rundown of those guidelines.

1. Avoid high-fat, high-calorie foods. You know why from reading preceding chapters. For your mind to be at its clearest and keenest, your brain must be richly supplied with blood, not losing it to the competition from your digestive system.
2. Eat protein first at lunch and dinner. It will switch on the alertness chemicals.
3. Avoid alcohol prior to work sessions. Just as important, drink none or very little (an ounce or less) at the cocktail hours, dinners, and other social events scheduled by the conference planners. Alcohol's sedative effect blurs the mind, impairing the ability to process information quickly and accurately and even to speak coherently. Since many of the most important business exchanges at a conference occur at off-hours gatherings, social drinking represents a very real professional hazard.
4. Drink just enough coffee or tea to maintain normal

caffeine levels in your body (by normal, of course, I mean *what is usual for you*). If you increase caffeine levels much above what you are accustomed to, you may find yourself feeling overstimulated and too distracted to concentrate and participate fully in the proceedings.

5. Use carbohydrate as a natural "sleeping pill" to help you unwind and relax at bedtime. Without it, you may remain too keyed up mentally and physically to fall asleep with ease. I don't have to tell you that without sufficient sleep you probably will feel groggy and unable to function at the top of your capabilities the following day.

Negotiating the Conference Breakfast

A common complaint at conferences has to do with the difficulty of ordering and eating breakfast in time to arrive punctually at the first working session of the day. As one of my clients complained to me recently, "It seems that no matter how early I get up, the hotel coffee shop already has a long line of people waiting to get in for breakfast. And room service is often so slow that I can't depend on getting my order filled before an early meeting. So what do I do? Go without eating, usually. Later on, at coffee break, I fill up on rolls, or I make up for my missed breakfast by eating twice as much as I should at lunch. There must be a better way."

Bring Your Own Breakfast

There *is* a better way. Slip a few simple breakfast foods into your overnight bag—or stop off for them on the way to the conference—and you will be able to have a nutritious morning meal at your leisure in your room at the hotel. A bring-it-yourself breakfast saves time and ensures that you will have enough in your stomach to tide you over until lunch. More important from the food/mind/mood point of view, it will help you avoid the kind of high-calorie, high-fat restaurant or catered breakfast that will, unless you pick and choose judiciously, bring you down with a jolt about midmorning.

Here's what to bring with you to the conference:

- Single-serving packages of instant hot or cold cereal, preferably a high-fiber brand that will satisfy part of your body's daily need for bulk or roughage
- Small boxes of raisins
- A pint or half-pint carton of low-fat milk or foil packs of powdered dry milk that can be converted with the addition of ice water into very acceptable whole skim milk*
- Rice cakes or Wasa bread wrapped in foil
- Containers of yogurt.* (Plain, vanilla, lemon, and coffee yogurt are lowest in calories.)
- Low-fat muffins, such as bran or corn muffins, or bagels, which are also low in fat. Keep them tightly wrapped in foil, and they will stay fresh for two or three days.
- Oranges, bananas, apples, or other fruit
- Juice, in boxes (lighter and less cumbersome than cans or bottles)
- Instant coffee (since jars are heavy, spoon some into a small plastic container or even a plastic food storage envelope) or tea bags
- An immersion heater
- A plastic cup and spoon

Naturally, you won't want to haul everything on the list above to a conference for a one-day stay. Shop and plan according to the duration of the conference.

The sample menus below illustrate how to combine the foods you bring along with you into nutritious breakfasts, low enough in calories and fat to prevent postmeal sluggishness and midmorning brain drain.

---

*If there is no refrigerator in your hotel room, keep milk and/or yogurt cold by placing them in an ice bucket—filled with ice, of course.

BRING-IT-YOURSELF MENU #1
1 4-ounce serving of juice or a piece of fruit
1 single-serving package of cold cereal or instant hot cereal
½ cup low-fat milk
1 corn or bran muffin, no butter
Coffee or tea (with low-fat milk, if you prefer)

BRING-IT-YOURSELF MENU #2
1 4-ounce serving of juice or a piece of fruit
1 8-ounce container of yogurt
1 bagel, rice cake, or Wasa bread with *no* butter
Coffee or tea (with low-fat milk, if you prefer)

A bring-it-yourself breakfast, as you can see, solves the problem of how to get enough of the right brain-powering food into your system in good time and without hassling with lines, crowds, and the temptation of high-fat, high-calorie breakfast specials listed on a menu. The drawback, of course, is that bringing your own breakfast requires some advance planning, shopping, and schlepping.

The Modified Continental Breakfast

I prefer to bring my own breakfasts to a conference, and I advise my clients to do the same. But there are other options. One alternative is to bring cereal only and augment it with the Continental breakfast available at many hotels simply by filling in an order card that hangs on the doorknob.

Items to check off on the card:

- Milk. Even if you don't use it in your coffee or tea, you can pour it on cereal.
- Juice or fruit
- Coffee or tea if you usually drink a caffeinated beverage in the morning
- Toast, a bagel, or muffin if available. You can eat any of these with your cereal as part of breakfast, or wrap and save for a late afternoon snack.

Do not order as part of your continental breakfast pastries such as croissants, doughnuts, sweet rolls, or Danish pastries. All are very high in fat and carbohydrate and supply little more in the way of nutrition than calories. (A croissant has about 200 calories; a Danish pastry somewhere between 250 and 300. A single-serving package of cereal supplies only about 70 calories. The difference is *fat.*) Not only that, but the high-calorie, high-fat pastries will linger in your stomach for hours, making you feel stuffed and sluggish of mind and body, the very opposite of the way you want to start out on conference mornings.

Restaurant and Catered Conference Breakfasts

Still another alternative, of course, is to brave the crowds and eat breakfast in the hotel dining room. Nothing wrong with that *if* you steel yourself and ignore the high-calorie, high-fat breakfast specials—the French toast and ham, the three-eggs-with-French-fries-and-bacon combinations, the corned beef hash with fried eggs, etc.—and adhere to the food/mood/mind guidelines that will maintain your peak mental performance during the first few hours of your day.

What should you order for your hotel conference breakfast? Essentially the same foods suggested for a bring-it-yourself morning meal:

* Half a grapefruit, cantaloupe, or four ounces of fruit juice
* Hot or cold cereal with low-fat milk (or if you are in the South, grits made without butter)
* Toast, a bagel, or a corn or bran muffin
* Coffee or tea, if you usually start the day with a shot of caffeine

For the cereal, you could substitute a cup of plain, coffee-, lemon-, or vanilla-flavored yogurt or a cup of low-fat cottage cheese. Another option would be to substitute two poached or soft-cooked eggs for the cereal, yogurt, or cottage cheese.

(Eat only the white of the second egg if you want to decrease cholesterol.)

Avoiding the Buffet Breakfast Hazard

A breakfast buffet can be a dazzlingly tempting obstacle course when your goal is to maintain morning mental alacrity, especially if breakfast is your favorite meal of the day. Obviously, it won't do to sample a little of everything.

One of my clients, a salesman for a computer software firm and a breakfast lover if ever there was one, came up with an ingenious way to sidestep the potential pitfalls of a breakfast buffet. He noticed something about the typical buffet spread that had escaped me until he pointed it out: The hot dishes and the cold foods are almost always grouped separately—the eggs Benedict, creamed chipped beef, bacon and sausages, and pancakes and crepes are segregated from the fruits, the cold cereals, the yogurt and cottage cheese, the muffins and bagels.

He is aware that almost everything in the hot foods section of a buffet table (with the exception of soft-boiled or poached eggs) will tend to undermine his ability to think clearly and quickly absorb new information, while most of the cold foods (pastries excepted) will enhance those same capabilities. So, he tells me, he simply strides determinedly—"and without looking"—past the hot dishes to the end of the table where the cold foods are located. "After all, I go to conferences to feed my mind, not my stomach," he says.

The A.M. Conference Coffee Break— Pass It Up

With a low-fat but highly nutritious and satisfying conference breakfast fueling your system, you shouldn't be hungry when coffee break is announced. And if you are not hungry, *don't* eat. Try not to be influenced by what your colleagues and co-conferees do—after all, *you* know the secret of enhancing mental alertness—no matter how enticingly the coffee break pastries are displayed.

There is only one instance in which it makes good sense from a brain-power point of view to waive the no-food rule at a conference coffee break. That is when you oversleep or miss breakfast for some other reason. When that happens, your hunger at midmorning may be intense enough to make you feel out-of-sorts, grumpy, even queasy. Thus some food at coffee break is definitely in order.

Nevertheless, don't fill up on pastries. Lunch is only a couple of hours away. Instead, have just enough of the lowest-fat, lowest-calorie food available to ease hunger pangs. Fruit of any kind is a good choice. If there is no fruit, choose an unbuttered bagel; an English, corn, or bran muffin; or a hard roll. All are lower in fat and therefore easier to digest than a croissant. For the same reason, if you must decide between plain coffee cake or a Danish pastry, take the coffee cake.

Caffeine at an A.M. Conference Coffee Break

As for coffee or tea, the guideline, as always is: If you are accustomed to drinking a caffeinated beverage at about this time each day, don't deviate from habit at a conference. It's important to keep caffeine at normal levels for you to prevent the potential discomfort—an energy slump, possibly even a headache!—of withdrawal.

Don't pour extra caffeine into your system, however, if you are not accustomed to it. You don't need it. If you want to sip something, have decaffeinated coffee or tea, fruit juice, seltzer, or plain water.

Conference Lunching for Greater Afternoon Effectiveness

What you eat at a conference lunch will affect directly your mental energy and motivation for hours afterward. Your food choices will influence your ability to take advantage of openings and opportunities and to participate vigorously and effectively in the afternoon sessions. It is not stretching the point to say that a good lunch, one that utilizes proven food/mind/mood principles, can make your entire day, while a bad lunch can break it.

You already know my guidelines for enhancing afternoon brain power: Eat a light, low-fat meal that is relatively high in protein and low in carbohydrates. Finish the protein component of your meal before you begin on the starch. Avoid alcohol.

Now let's look at how you can apply these guidelines in three special conference contexts.

The Do-It-Yourself Lunch

Just as my personal preference, based on my experiences at dozens of conferences all over the world, is to assemble my own breakfast from foods I pack and take along to the meeting, I am equally partial to putting together my own lunch whenever it is feasible. It saves me the time I otherwise would spend waiting to be served in a hotel dining room or restaurant, time I prefer to use for running or other physical activity. Just as important, of course, is that when I am in control of my own lunch menu, I know that I will be getting exactly the food I need to work hard, long, and better during the afternoon.

To illustrate, let me tell you about a meeting on obesity that I attended just a few months ago. It was held in Switzerland. The hotel and conference center, next door to each other, were both on beautiful Lake Geneva. Along the shore of the lake is a large park with several miles of footpaths. Knowing about this sylvan setting in advance, I decided to break up the long days of sitting, note-taking, and speechmaking with lunch hour runs in the park, followed by smallish, high-protein, low-fat meals—the kind that can be eaten and digested quickly—in my room.

On the first day of the meeting, I went to a small grocery store near the conference center and bought four-ounce "pop-top" cans of water-packed tuna, some carrots, celery, oranges, and yogurt. Since my hotel room was typically European, in that it was equipped with a small refrigerator, storage was not a problem. Breakfast was brought to the room Swiss-style, and I saved a fresh roll from that meal to eat at lunch each day.

As soon as we broke at midday, I zipped up to my room, changed into shorts and running shoes, jogged for half an hour, then zipped back to a lunch of tuna, raw vegetables, a roll, and yogurt for dessert.

By the time the conference got underway again after lunch, guess who was feeling fit, full of energy, and eager to plunge into the work of the afternoon? Right! I'm sorry to have to report that although the subject of this conference was obesity, many of the experts, tops in their field, returned from lunch seemingly sluggish, slowed-down, and unfocused—exhibiting, in other words, the unmistakable effects of a heavy meal and its consequences, digestive overload.

I am aware that many American hotel rooms are not equipped with refrigerators and that you cannot depend on fresh rolls being delivered each morning to be saved and eaten at lunch. That doesn't mean you can't have a mentally energizing, brain-powering lunch in your room at midday . . . plus half an hour or so of "free" time to refresh yourself with a walk, a run, some simple calisthentics, or a quick workout in the hotel health club.

When you pack for the conference, be sure to take with you an immersion heater, a collapsible mug, a can opener, and plastic spoons and forks (or save a spoon and fork if you order from room service). In addition, bring along or shop on your arrival for the following:

- A small can of water-packed tuna
- A small can of boned, cooked chicken

- A small can of sardines, packed in tomato or mustard sauce, not oil
- Packets of breadsticks, whole-grain crackers, rice cakes, or other unsweetened crackers
- A package of small pita rounds. (If you keep the plastic bag tightly closed, bread will stay fresh for days.)
- Soup-in-a-cup mixes. (Look for low-salt varieties if you must restrict sodium.)
- Fruit: a banana, an orange, strawberries, blueberries. (See if you can find some that are grown locally.)
- Carrots, red or green peppers
- Half-pint (one cup) containers of cottage cheese and yogurt. (These can be kept chilled in an ice bucket.)

From these few items you can make the following mind-motivating conference lunches:

DO-IT-YOURSELF CONFERENCE LUNCH #1
1 small can water-packed tuna on pita bread
1 carrot and 1 red or green pepper, sliced
1 envelope onion soup-in-a-cup mix
1 banana and handful of raisins

DO-IT-YOURSELF CONFERENCE LUNCH #2
1 small can boned, cooked chicken
3 rice cakes
1 envelope tomato soup-in-a-cup mix
1 cup plain yogurt, topped with
½ cup sliced berries

DO-IT-YOURSELF CONFERENCE LUNCH #3
1 small can sardines in tomato or mustard sauce
3 breadsticks or 1 pita bread
1 envelope chicken soup-in-a-cup mix
1 cup cottage cheese (buy pineapple-flavored, if you like the taste), topped with
1 orange, sectioned, and handful of raisins

The Catered Conference Lunch

There is one thing you can always count on when the conference lunch is catered: You will be served more food than your digestive organs can deal with quickly and efficiently—so much food, in fact, that if you eat it all, your major activity in the hours that follow will be digestion.

If you read our chapters on working meals and preperformance eating, however, you will be able to cope.

Limit the amount of protein you consume to about four ounces, which probably will be anywhere from one-third to one-half less than you are served, since caterers supply between six and eight ounces of meat, chicken, or fish per person. (Because you won't have a food scale with you, you should know ahead of time approximately what four ounces of protein looks like. As I mentioned earlier, practice makes perfect and the best way to learn how to gauge a four-ounce portion by sight is to weigh your food at home and/or spend time in a supermarket looking at the packaged and weighed beef, chicken, fish, etc.)

Once you have eaten your four ounces of protein, you can begin the rest of your meal. Caterers usually figure on about one cup of rice or a medium potato per person, amounts that are safe in terms of not overloading your digestive organs. But do not eat the starchy component of your conference lunch if it is drenched with butter or swimming in a rich sauce. Have an unbuttered roll or slice of bread instead.

Salad and vegetables are safe, too, unless richly sauced or dressed. If possible, notify your waiter before salad and vegetables are served that you want yours plain. If he can't accommodate you, see if you can pick your way through pieces covered with sauce or oil and eat those that aren't. If *that* is impossible, don't eat the salad or vegetables.

Dessert? *Don't eat it unless it is fruit*.

Coffee? Yes, if you normally have some at lunch or feel the

need of a shot of instant brain stimulation. I often have noticed that the more prestigious the conference and the higher in status the conferees, the more counterproductive the meal is, in the sense that it prevents the VIPs from achieving what they presumably hoped to accomplish.

A scientific meeting at which almost everyone present was on the cutting edge of research in her or his own specialized field was held in Europe at a three-star hotel known for its elegant suites and sumptuous cuisine. Lunch started with a fish mousse and proceeded to a meat course of veal with an exquisite sauce, an assortment of vegetables, buttered and sprigged with parsley, and potatoes, also sauced. Then there was a salad course, followed by a huge cheese section. The meal ended with an assortment of mousses and petit fours.

I heard about it from my co-conferees. You see, I stayed away from this eating extravaganza in order to get in some running and afterward had a simple meal in my room. But I know from on-the-spot observation the effects of that grand lunch on the others. At the beginning of the afternoon session, most of the participants shuffled in as though they had lead in their shoes—and their stomachs—then slumped down in their chairs. When the lights went out for a slide presentation, so did they.

Conference Lunching at Cafeteria or Restaurant

Of course, not all conference lunches are on a par with the splendid spread I have just described. In fact, more often than not, you, as attendee, will be required to find your own meal, either at an on-site cafeteria, coffee shop or snack bar (if the conference is held at a university, convention center, or corporate headquarters), or at a nearby restaurant.

Unlike catered lunches in a hotel dining room, where the menu has been planned down to the last bite, a cafeteria or restaurant lunch allows you some freedom of choice. Keep these guidelines in mind as you make your selection:

- Do not choose as a main course any dish that does not contain obvious, discernible protein—pieces or chunks of chicken, beef, fish, or shellfish. (I am reminded here of the cafeteria food at a large Midwestern university-sponsored conference. The main courses that day were a broccoli and cheese casserole; a brown rice, raisin, and cheese casserole; and a fruit salad covered with something resembling mayonnaise. Any of these would have had me nodding out after the lunch break. None contained more than negligible amounts of protein, and all were high in fat. Luckily, I found some cottage cheese almost hidden among the greens at the salad bar and filled up on that source of protein.)
- Usually okay are main dish salads such as tuna, chicken, or shrimp salad or a cold meat or chef's salad. But look them over before you make a final choice (these items are usually on display in a cafeteria) to make sure that the protein is not obscured by a heavy mayonnaise dressing. If mayo seems to be the main ingredient in these salads, pick something else. Main dish salads often have a scoop of potato salad or macaroni salad on the side. If you want your brain to stay quick and agile throughout the afternoon sessions, don't eat them. Instead, choose a lower-fat form of carbohydrate, such as an unbuttered roll or one or two slices of plain bread.
- Any clear soup, as well as vegetable, meat, or chicken soup (assuming they're not too fatty) is safe. But creamed soups, bisques, and creamy chowders (New England- or Boston-style) are too rich and heavy if you want to function after lunch at the peak of your mental powers.
- Sandwiches made with lean beef, lean ham, turkey, or chicken are good protein choices. So is a plain hamburger minus cheese and French fries.
- Fruits and vegetables—assuming that they are neither heavily buttered, sauced, or mayonnaised—are mind/mood neutral in that they neither enhance nor detract

from mental acuity. Eat them in moderation—no more than one and a half to two cups.

I am always as specific as I can be in recommending what to eat to enhance the brain power of those I counsel. So here are lunches readily available in conference site cafeterias, coffee shops, and non-specialty restaurants. They have helped dozens of my conference-going clients. They can boost your postlunch potential, too.

CONFERENCE LUNCH MENU #1—CAFETERIA

1 serving chicken, fish, or lean beef (baked, grilled, or roasted, not fried; ask server to hold any sauce or gravy)
1 serving plain steamed rice
1 serving each green and bright-colored vegetables, unbuttered, *or* 1 serving salad and 1 serving bright-colored vegetable
1 serving fruit, unsweetened
1 cup low-fat milk (optional)
Coffee or tea as usual

CONFERENCE LUNCH MENU #2—CAFETERIA

1 cup clear soup
1 pack saltines
1 container plain, vanilla, or lemon-flavored yogurt
1 serving fruit, unsweetened
Coffee or tea as usual

CONFERENCE LUNCH MENU #3—FAST-FOOD RESTAURANT

1 quarter-pound hamburger with roll, no cheese or sauce
1 serving salad, made with carrots, green and red pepper, spinach, broccoli or cauliflower (most fast-food restaurants now have salad bars). Dress *very* lightly with vinegar and oil.
1 cup low-fat milk (optional)
Coffee or tea as usual

CONFERENCE LUNCH MENU #4—COFFEE SHOP

1 chicken, turkey, or lean roast beef sandwich with lettuce and tomato on whole-wheat or pita bread (with mustard or ketchup if desired, no mayonnaise)

1 serving fruit, unsweetened
1 cup low-fat milk (optional)
Coffee or tea as usual

As you will notice, the conference lunch menus above are hearty enough to see you through to the end of the last working session of the day free of the debilitating effects of hunger. Although it is important to avoid eating the *wrong* foods, it is almost as important to eat enough of the *right* foods. Otherwise, you may be tempted to "pig out" at the coffee break.

The Afternoon Conference Coffee Break

As I explained in the first part of this book, there is a tendency in late afternoon for your body's internal clock to begin signaling that it is time to start winding down for the day. But it is important to your professional advancement to stay mentally awake and vigorous until the last moments of the last session of the day.

Once again, food will do it for you.

- If you are feeling hungry (not likely, if you ate enough for lunch), try to find some low-fat protein to eat. Probably the best you can hope for now is plain yogurt or cottage cheese. Four ounces of either will assist your brain to make more of the alertness chemicals.
- Do *not* eat cheese, peanuts, peanut butter, or other protein foods that are high in fat.
- If there are no protein foods available but you want something safe to eat, have fruit or fruit juice.
- Avoid at all costs starchy and sweet foods, including soft drinks that are sweetened with sugar. Even one or two ounces of these foods will put a damper on mental energy and alertness.
- Pour yourself a cup of coffee or tea if you are a moderate

drinker of these beverages and it has been several hours since your last cup. If you are a heavy coffee or tea drinker, you probably will need more caffeine now to maintain your normal caffeine levels. Otherwise drink water, seltzer, or club soda.

Carbohydrate Cravers' Alert!

If the results of the food/mind/mood test in chapter 4 indicate that you are a carbohydrate craver, *disregard the above,* and eat an ounce or two of something sweet or starchy at coffee break time. Carbohydrate now will prevent the restlessness, irritability, boredom, and loss of concentration that are the result of serotonin levels dropping too low. If you have already begun to feel edgy and unfocused, it will quickly restore your mind and your mood.

Since typical coffee break snacks tend to be too high in fat to give quick, sure results, be prepared. Stow in your brief-case or bag something you can eat quietly (in case you need your carbohydrate fix in the middle of an afternoon meeting). Small packages of gumdrops, jelly beans, licorice bits, or miniature marshmallows are good choices. (The candy doesn't need to be unwrapped once the package is opened.) If noise is not a consideration, a small package of cookies or crackers (four to six in a pack) would be ideal.

If you didn't come prepared and the carbohydrates available at coffee break are all too high in fat to do you immediate good, have a regular soft drink (not sugar-free), or pour a cup of coffee or tea and mix in two to three teaspoons of sugar.

The Predinner Snack— Your Opportunity to Unwind

So far in this what-to-eat guide for getting more out of conference-going, I have been urging you to go easy on carbohydrates (unless, of course, you are a carbohydrate craver) because of their potential to calm you, relax you, and bring on feelings of drowsiness. I don't have to remind you that these low-key states are not conducive to active participation or to quick and efficient processing of information, new ideas, and techniques.

But when the last session of the day has ended and you return to your room, or perhaps linger on to spend a social hour or two with colleagues and new friends, carbohydrates become the foods of choice. They'll help your brain come down from its high-energy levels and allow you to leave the stresses of the day behind.

My own experiences as a conference-goer have taught me that the last session of the day usually ends about ninety minutes after the midafternoon coffee break. *Then* it is time to relax and recoup.

Since you have been limiting carbohydrate intake in order to maintain a state of high mental energy and alertness, by late afternoon your body will be especially hungry for the tranquilizing effects of a sweet or starchy food. In fact, you may feel such a strong desire for carbohydrates now that you find yourself heading automatically toward the newsstand or snack bar in search of cookies or candy. Look around and you probably will see many of your fellow conferees doing the same.

Alcohol, too, can be an aid to relaxation, and no doubt most of the conference-goers who don't take a carbohydrate break after the last meeting of the day, will take an alcohol break instead.

However, if you must be alert and articulate throughout the dinner hour, I am going to insist that you avoid alcohol now and unwind with carbohydrate. It will calm, compose, and refocus your mind simply by activating the production of the natural brain chemical serotonin. Alcohol, on the other hand, will relax you, but at a cost. You may be *so* relaxed and unfocused during the dinner, reception, and/or after-dinner meeting to come that you are unable to demonstrate the keenness of mind and quick grasp of facts and concepts that mark you as a winner.

My clients who have tried both alcohol and carbohydrate for predinner relaxation concede that carbohydrate is the superior tranquilizer when they must perform mentally through and after dinner.

For example, one of my clients is required to promote her company's ideas and products at frequent sales conferences. She is under considerable pressure, since her meetings often begin at 8 A.M. and last until 6 P.M., after which she is expected to continue to make contacts and keep up the sales pitch at dinner. She came to me because she was beginning to feel she lacked the motivation necessary to do her best at these conferences. "It looks as though I may have to consider a slower-paced and less demanding job," she confided.

I asked how she recouped in the hours after meetings and before dinner. "I head for the bar and practically gulp down a Bloody Mary," she said. "Then I order a second one from room service and sip it as I shower, change, and do my makeup. I suppose I'm not *really* a drinker, though," she added, "because I feel numb for the remainder of the evening."

My advice to her, of course, was to switch from alcohol to a carbohydrate snack during the postmeeting, predinner interval. I gave her a list of choices. She was delighted when she saw that vanilla wafers, her favorite cookie when she was a child, was one of them.

Weeks later she reported back: "After afternoon meetings now, I return immediately to my room, stretch out on the bed, turn on the TV—it doesn't matter which program; I don't actually watch—and have five or six vanilla wafers and a cup of mint tea with sugar. Fifteen minutes later I feel calm and content as a pussycat, with not a care in the world.

"Then," she went on, "about an hour after my snack I shower, get dressed, and feel ready to take on the world again—not fuzzed out as I used to be when I relaxed with Bloody Marys. It's truly amazing. I take vanilla wafers to every conference now."

The only possible drawback to having a carbohydrate snack after a day of conference meetings is that if you must shift into high mental gear within forty-five minutes or so of eating, you may still be experiencing the relaxing effects of your snack when you should be back in a state of full mental alert. This is rarely a problem, though. At most conferences you will have more than enough time to snack and enjoy the tranquilizing effect of carbohydrate in the time between the last meeting of the day and dinner or other evening commitments.

You may even be able to get a few moments of sleep. If you *can* nap, do so. You'll feel even more refreshed and mentally invigorated afterward.

Postmeeting, Predinner Conference Relaxers

One to one and one-half ounces of almost any starchy or sweet food will have the desired relaxation effect. However, in working with clients, and through my own personal experience, I have discovered that the following snacks are especially useful in inducing tranquility and composure:

- Gumdrops
- Jelly beans (and other "jelly" candies, such as Chuckles)
- Granola bars
- Peanut butter crackers
- Plain or cream-filled chocolate cookies that come wrapped four to six in a package
- Pretzels and popcorn (usually available in one-and-a-half-ounce bags)
- A bagel or a muffin, a miniature pita loaf lightly spread with peanut butter, or rice cakes (from your personal store of food, if you brought some of your own, as I suggested earlier in this chapter)

Conference Dinners:
When They Matter and When They Don't

"Off-Duty" Conference Dinners

When you know for sure that the last afternoon session of your conference day will also be the last *working* session of the day, what you eat for dinner becomes relatively unimportant. Since you won't need to be concerned with performing and participating at the top of your mental capabilities during your meal or after it, you may as well order what you like for dinner and enjoy.

My only caveat with regard to the off-duty conference dinner has to do with calories. You don't need to worry if you are string-bean skinny. Eat up. But if your weight is just about right and you want it to stay that way or if you are at all over your ideal weight, you probably should exercise some restraint. After all, in most conference settings the opportunity for *other* types of exercise are few and far between. I've seen it happen to clients and colleagues: A few huge, *fattening* off-duty conference dinners that were not offset by a half hour or so of vigorous activity each day caused the pounds to pile on with breathtaking rapidity. (A fellow M.I.T. researcher gained five pounds in as many days at her last conference!)

You can easily keep calories within reasonable limits at off-duty conference dinners if you simply remember—and act on—a few basic points of fact.

An average alcoholic drink supplies approximately 100 calories. A tablespoon of salad dressing, sour cream, or butter also delivers about 100 calories. Deep- or batter-fried foods will have in the neighborhood of 100 calories more than the average four- to six-ounce serving of the same food grilled, roasted, or boiled. You can shave 300, 400, or more calories from your evening meal just by having seltzer or mineral water instead of an alcoholic drink, by going easy on—or avoiding completely—salad dressing, sour cream, and/or butter, and by ordering your food grilled, roasted, or boiled.

Select your restaurant for the evening with calories in mind. Oriental food—Chinese and Japanese—tends to be far lower in calories than most of the foods offered in Italian, French, Mexican, and other ethnic restaurants, and in steakhouses and other eateries indigenous to the United States, the exception being places that specialize in seafood. (Broiled fish or plain-cooked shellfish are always excellent low-calorie choices.) By all means, avoid any restaurant that appeals to its customers on the basis of quantity of food served rather than quality.

"On-Duty" Conference Dinners

Off-duty conference dinners, in which a group of colleagues and newfound conference friends decide to go out for an evening of sociability and relaxation, have a way of turning into on-duty dinners. Be sensitive to this fact. What happens and doesn't happen in the hours spent sharing a purely social meal can have more of an impact in terms of contacts made, points confirmed, and transactions settled than whole days in a meeting room discussing official business. Therefore, unless you will be dining with friends who are in no way connected with the conference you are attending, it usually is wise to eat so as to keep your wits about you, so that you can take advantage of any new information or opportunities to advance your own or your company's interests.

One of my clients learned this lesson for himself, to his great chagrin and embarrassment. This man, a rising star in a highly esoteric scientific field, told me that since he worked so hard for so many daytime hours at the conferences he attended, he felt justified in giving himself permission to eat whatever struck his fancy at dinner. One evening, he and several colleagues who worked with him at the same research facility decided to dine at a highly recommended French restaurant located near the conference center. One of his colleagues brought along a newcomer. "I didn't know him from Adam," my client commented ruefully. "But it turned out that this fellow was in a *very* senior position at the private foundation evaluating my latest grant proposal."

Although he may be mistaken after all, my client is convinced that if he hadn't eaten himself almost into a stupor—and in consequence essentially ignored the newcomer and the conversation when it eventually turned to research—his project might have had a better chance of being approved for funding. "But no such luck. I blew it," he sighed.

Of course, he is aware that luck has little to do with it. And in the future he is determined to be cautious about what he eats and drinks at any off-duty conference dinner. Often, there is a hidden agenda in these sociable get-togethers.

As for those official on-duty receptions and dinners, when the agenda is anything but hidden, it is *imperative* to eat in ways that enhance brain power and mental alertness.

Let's review the most important dos and don'ts to help you maintain peak mental capacity during both off-duty conference dinners when business might creep into the conversation and frankly business-related receptions and dinners.

- Do not have predinner cocktails or more than one glass of wine during dinner. The lateness of the hour will increase the capacity of alcohol to make you feel drowsy, tipsy, or both. If you are thirsty or feel naked without a glass in your hand or something in your wineglass at the table, ask for plain water, seltzer, or mineral water with a twist of lemon or lime.
- Don't eat carbohydrate before protein.
- Do eat a protein appetizer if one is available. Good examples: shrimp cocktail, smoked salmon, oysters, marinated mussels, smoked duck, tiny meatballs.
- If there are no protein hors d'oeuvres or appetizers, delay eating until the protein part of your meal is served. Have the protein first, then go on to the carbohydrates.

- Portion sizes will be generous, so eat only one-third to one-half of your entrée. Ask to have yours served plain. If that is impossible, try to eat around any sauce.
- Keep fat intake low by eating salad without dressing, and vegetables, potato, or rice unbuttered and unsauced. If these items come to the table already drenched in a rich dressing or sauce, eat one or two mouthfuls but no more.
- Do not have dessert unless it is plain, unsweetened fruit, unadorned with whipped cream or liqueur.
- Don't finish a conference banquet with coffee or tea *unless* you are to be the after-dinner speaker or are scheduled to participate in a postdinner discussion and you think you will need some quick mental stimulation to carry you through.

By now I'm sure you know the principles of eating to maintain brain power during and after a conference dinner or banquet. They are the same principles that will keep you motivated and mentally energetic in almost any demanding situation. In summing up, keep in mind that *the overall premises upon which these guidelines are based are more important than specific food suggestions*.

In following the guidelines you will have to do some discreet picking and choosing at restaurants or at catered dinners and receptions. But if you adhere to these suggestions just once in circumstances that are mentally strenuous, I know you will be so pleased with the boost in your performance potential that you will want to make eating for better brain power a permanent part of your life.

A personal anecdote may be in order here: Since I practice what I preach—because it has worked for me time and again—I often find myself one of the few in a room who are still alert and eager to participate after a long conference meal.

I remember one banquet in particular. The menu was a magnificent example of mentally counterproductive food planning: high in carbohydrates, fat, calories, and wine and lowish in protein (the entrée consisted of heavily sauced but small pieces of veal), with a vanilla soufflé topped with chocolate sauce for dessert. After the meal, there were several short speeches introducing the new president and vice-presidents of the organization sponsoring the conference. Finally, the keynote speaker was announced. I looked around, hearing the gentle but unmistakable sound of snoring. At every table, eyelids were drooping and heads nodding.

As it turned out, the speaker was excellent. But I'm afraid that only I and one or two others in the audience were wide awake enough to appreciate his eloquence and to hear his ingenious new approach to a problem all of us were concerned with.

Snacks for Sleeping

If there is *any* drawback in the brain-powering eating techniques I have been advocating here, it lies in the difficulties you may experience when the time comes to turn off the mental energy you have been maintaining and fall rapidly into deep sleep at bedtime.

But even that potential problem has a quick and easy food solution. Simply eat one to one and one-half ounces of low-fat carbohydrate between fifteen and thirty minutes before you slip into bed, as noted at the beginning of this chapter.

10. Conference Planners' Confidential

Even if you already have been the organizing force behind many meetings—whether they lasted for half a day or ran for almost a week or more—you may be unaware of the critical role played by the meals you arrange to serve to attendees.

I am not exaggerating when I say that conference food can make or break an entire meeting, just as it will enhance or detract from the performance of the individual conference-goer.

As an example of what I'm talking about, let me tell you about a client who works in the insurance industry. Her job requires that she attend a conference each month on average, sometimes two. She knows and adheres to my guidelines and strategies and has told me many times that the food/mind/ mood principles have given her the edge she needs to quickly pick up and adapt new ideas, make new contacts, and otherwise use conference time to her and her company's advantage.

But she often has been frustrated by the behavior of her fellow conference-goers. "I look around the room during meetings and see them sprawled in their chairs, doodling on notepads, daydreaming, yawning, sometimes even dozing off after lunch. Their input is minimal, their enthusiasm nil, and this can't help but affect negatively the go-getters who came to meetings eager to learn, trade information, and turn leads into money-making opportunities."

A recent conference experience, she said, was amazingly different. The agenda was a nutrition-related one, and the conference planners must have felt honor-bound to offer healthy meals. Everything was low in fat, with plain roasted, grilled, or baked chicken, fish, or meat for lunch and dinner. The vegetables were flavored with herbs and spices instead of sauce or butter. And desserts were almost always fruit—either stewed or fresh fruit salad, or poached pears, baked apples, or fresh fruit sorbets. Even the coffee breaks were planned to keep attendees on their toes: Instead of pastries, sweet rolls, and croissants, there were bran muffins, yogurt, and an assortment of fruit.

"I was struck by the amount of energy in the room after lunch on the first day. Instead of sitting blank-faced and bored, people had their hands up, asking questions. They were debating points made by the speaker. They were actively involved. It was very, very stimulating."

I can't promise that in following my meal planning suggestions, you, as conference organizer, automatically will create a livelier, more intellectually stimulating environment . . . or that your speakers will all give sparkling presentations . . . or even that attendees will listen, respond, and participate with greater enthusiasm. But I can promise that if you plan conference menus with these food/mind/mood strategies in mind, you will increase dramatically the chances that your meeting will be a valuable and productive event for all involved.

Cardinal Rules of
Conference Menu Planning

Less Is More

Conferees will feel more energetic, more attentive, and more motivated if you underfeed them. No, I am not suggesting that you give them starvation rations, only that you plan meals large enough to satisfy hunger but not so large that those who feel obliged to clean their plates will come away from the table feeling stuffed.

By feeding your guests frugally, you will be helping to prevent the lethargy, loginess, and brain drain that inevitably result from overeating. Thus, if you are in charge of planning conference meals, your first order of business is to see to it that portion sizes are modest and that the calorie count of meals is not excessive.

The guidelines that follow are necessarily approximate. (It is almost impossible to plan a meal, or even a single dish, to conform to a precise calorie count; there are too many variables with regard to ingredients, seasonings, cuts of meat used, etc.) Nevertheless, these pointers should help you and/or the caterer you will be working with put together menus for meals that are adequate but not too heavy or high in calories.

PORTION SIZES. Conference planners tend to be overly generous with food, partly, no doubt, because they don't want to appear to be skimping and partly because they want conferees to feel satisfied and well taken care of during their stay. It is not unusual, for example, for meat portions to be in excess of ten ounces!

Hardly anyone but a professional wrestler needs that much food at one sitting (and certainly not conference-goers who will spend most of their time doing nothing more strenuous than pushing a pen), and paying for it is a waste of money.

What *are* the ideal portion sizes for conference meals? Breakfast aside (conference-goers often serve themselves from a buffet table or get their own breakfast from room service or a coffee shop at the convention site), plan on serving the following amounts:

	LUNCH
Protein	4–5 ounces
Starch (rice, potatoes, etc.)	3/4 cup or 1 potato; 1 roll
Vegetables	3/4 cup cooked, plus 1 cup salad
Dessert	1 piece fruit, 1 cup fruit salad, or 1 cup sorbet

	DINNER
Protein	5–6 ounces
Starch (rice, potatoes, etc.)	3/4–1 cup or 1 potato; 1 roll
Vegetables	3/4 cup cooked, plus 1 cup salad
Dessert	1 piece fruit, 1 cup fruit salad, or 1 cup sorbet

CALORIES. Calorie requirements, of course, differ from person to person, so it is impossible to pinpoint the exact number of calories per meal that would increase the mental potential of each and every conference-goer. However, since we know for a fact that too many calories take the edge off mental sharpness, it is possible to arrive at an approximate maximum number of calories . . . and hope that those men and women who need fewer than the maximum will eat proportionately less.

• *Plan lunch menus that supply each person with about 500–600 calories.*

• *For dinner, figure on approximately 600–800 calories per person.*

In making your calculations, be sure to include everything on the menu—from hors d'oeuvres to appetizer to soup to entrée, salad, side dishes, and dessert.

Keep It Low in Fat

There is no mystery to planning reduced-fat meals. You probably already know the principles. But here are simple reminders:

- Roast or grill instead of frying.
- Choose chicken, fish, or other seafood over red meat.
- If your conference runs for more than a day or so and you feel you must include at least one meal featuring red meat, have veal or lean beef instead of fresh pork, ham, or lamb.
- Serve vegetables plain, preferably steamed, without butter or sauce.
- Plan on clear, fat-free soups—never creamy soups or bisques.
- Avoid dishes that have mayonnaise as a major ingredient, as well as those made with hard cheese or cheese sauce.
- For dessert, serve fruit as often as possible. Sorbet is a good second choice. Plain cake is preferable to cake with a buttery icing. Worst choices: cream pies, cheesecake, creamy puddings, and pastries made with large amounts of butter or shortening.

Start Meals with Protein

As you know from this book, protein spurs production of dopamine and norepinephrine, the alertness chemicals, which will keep conference-goers feeling motivated and mentally wide awake. Proteins also block the manufacture of serotonin, the calming chemical, which relaxes and, as the day progresses, tends to create feelings of sluggishness and/or drowsiness in the eater.

How can you be sure that conferees will get protein into their systems before they begin to eat carbohydrates?

Arrange to have a protein appetizer or first course. Possibilities include shrimp cocktail, cold curried fish or chicken, smoked salmon, clams on the half-shell, oysters, tiny meat-balls, raw vegetables with a yogurt dip, seafood chowder (but not the creamy New England variety), or a meat or chicken soup. Your caterer will have more ideas. Don't serve bread, breadsticks, or rolls until after this first protein course has been cleared away.

Plan to Serve Proteins and/or High-Fiber Carbohydrates at Breaks.

Protein foods are the snacks of choice at the traditional ten-thirty and three-thirty between-meeting breaks, for the same reason that they should be served and eaten first at meals.

The only problem is that, with the exception of cottage cheese and yogurt, there are few protein snacks that are both inexpensive enough not to break your conference budget and suitable for quick and easy eating. Herring tidbits, chunks of chicken or crabmeat, smoked oysters, etc., are all more or less pricey and require plates, forks, and/or knives for serving. Hard-boiled eggs are cheaper and less difficult to serve, but many conference-goers may have had them for breakfast. And because eggs are so high in cholesterol, it is not wise to encourage people to eat them in unlimited quantities.

If protein foods are problematic at breaks, what's the alternative?

Provide carbohydrate foods that are high in fiber and low in fat.

To understand why high-fiber carbohydrates are better at preventing mental slow-down than low- or no-fiber carbohydrates, you must first be aware that low-fiber carbohydrates such as breads, rolls, and pastries cause an almost instant elevation in blood sugar levels and a correspondingly quick and large release of insulin from the pancreas to deal with the sugar. This sudden release of large amounts of insulin ulti-mately stimulates production of serotonin, with all its mind-lulling potential.

Essentially the same sequence of physiological events occurs when a high-fiber carbohydrate food is eaten. But there is a major and important difference: The fiber decreases significantly the speed with which nutrients are digested and pass into the bloodstream. As a result, insulin is released more gradually, and smaller amounts of tryptophan enter the brain at a much slower rate.

The effects of slowed-down serotonin manufacture are not as dramatic or intense as an immediate upsurge of this chemical. Thus, conference-goers will not experience the same abrupt loss of motivation and brain power when they eat high-fiber carbohydrates that they would if they ate low- or no-fiber carbohydrates.

Carbohydrates that are rich in fiber and thus slower to act include such foods as bran muffins, fruit and nut mixtures (such as trail mix), and roasted chickpeas and soybeans—all fairly high in fiber. Other good between-session snack choices are rice cakes, dried fruit, and "fruit" or "vegetable" bread made with whole-wheat flour, oat bran, and apples, bananas, pumpkin, or zucchini.

Make Alcohol Hard to Come By

Regardless of the initial stimulating effect of alcohol, it is inevitably sedating. And obviously, people in a semisedated state will not participate enthusiastically. For this reason, think long and hard about whether you really want to have wine, beer, or cocktails at cocktail lunches.

Alcohol at conference dinners is less detrimental. Unless there will be after-dinner speeches and/or working sessions, most of the official business of the day will be over with by the time conference-goers gather for the meal.

However, keep in mind that much unofficial business is transacted during and after dinner. It is often a time when debatable points made earlier are discussed and clarified and valuable inside information is traded and professional contacts consolidated. Thus, I believe it is important to limit the availability of alcohol even this late in the day.

If you opt to make alcohol hard to come by, as I suggest, you must make sure that there are ample liquid alternatives for thirsty guests. Waiters should be instructed to keep water glasses filled at all times, and the paying bar at receptions and dinners should be well stocked with plenty of lower-priced nonalcoholic beverages such as mineral water, seltzer, fruit juices, and soft drinks.

There will always be conferees who have little interest in the proceedings and for whom the meals, receptions, and after-meeting social events are the main reason for attending. They will be displeased, if not irate, at the lack of readily available alcohol. But by making them seek out their drinks rather than allowing the liquor to flow freely, you can ensure their greater participation—perhaps despite themselves. Remember, you are not planning the conference as an opportunity for attendees to break with routine and party for a few days, but to accomplish certain objectives. Steel yourself for grumbling and complaints—and after the conference, be prepared for compliments on how well-organized and productive it all was!

Have Caffeinated and Noncaffeinated Beverages Available at Meals and Breaks

Caffeine, as you know from this book, is an excellent *and necessary* aid to mental clarity, accuracy, and energy for those who are accustomed to drinking coffee or tea daily.

When people who are habituated to a certain amount of caffeine experience a sudden cutoff in their daily dosage, dramatically reduced brain power and slowed responses may be the result.

I witnessed a rather startling demonstration of how caffeine deprivation can interfere with mental performance several years ago at a conference in Europe. The setting couldn't have been lovelier: an ancient chateau out in the countryside, many miles from the nearest town. The isolation seemed ideal at first, since it would force the conference participants to stay on the grounds and work, work, work, with a little time out for socializing in the evenings.

However, halfway through the first day it became apparent that something had gone disastrously wrong. After lunch, many of the conference-goers—myself included—felt too fatigued to think, and some even fell asleep. It was not the food; it was the absence of coffee. Although it had been served in the early morning, at breakfast, our conference planner neglected to make it available at the midmorning break and at lunch gave us a choice of mineral water or wine but no caffeinated beverage.

Many of us were still sleepy and jet-lagged from our transatlantic flight the day before, and this combination—lack of sleep and lack of caffeine—was so soporific that the meeting scheduled for just after lunch was a total waste. It was obvious to the conference planner that immediate steps had to be taken. There were hushed whisperings among members of the sponsoring group, a scurrying among the staff; a car was dispatched to the town, and within an hour or so it came speeding back up the long, winding drive, whereupon a coffee break was announced.

Because of the tremendous variation in the need for and tolerance of caffeine, you must see to it that noncaffeinated beverages are also available at meals and breaks. Thus, your conference-planning food list should include along with regular coffee and tea, a supply of good decaffeinated coffee and tea, herb tea, seltzer and mineral water, fruit juices, and a selection of soft drinks, including sugar-free and caffeine-free varieties.

As alternatives to these more traditional beverages, you might also want to consider serving, as they do on cruise ships, such unexpected but usually much appreciated beverages as hot consommé, bouillon, or, if the weather is warm, fruit frappes, refreshing gazpacho, or a cold fruit soup such as iced sour cherry soup. Hot and cold soups are easy to serve. They have no sugar (except for the fruit soups, which contain only natural fructose, a form of sugar that does not signal the brain suddenly to increase serotonin production). Just as important, they are fat-free and won't contribute to digestive overload. It's definitely worth giving them a try.

Have Courage . . . and Be Firm

The conference food guidelines outlined here *will* make a difference. They will increase the motivation, enthusiasm, mental accuracy, and energy of the participants—but only if you put them into practice.

If you plan mixed menus that allow conference-goers a choice between the heavy, high-fat, high-calorie foods most of them have come to expect at professional meetings and the lighter, lower-fat, lower-calorie meals that I recommend, chances are that many of them will select the former.

It's to be expected. Few people know that pastries at midmorning break will cause serotonin production to skyrocket, immediately making participants feel less energetic and more inclined to go off into a daydream.

They won't know that they can expect better participation from all for several hours afterward if they start lunch with a protein food, avoid alcohol, and have a light, low-fat entrée followed by fruit for dessert. They won't know that cookies and cake at the afternoon break will lead to mental and physical lethargy, or that a cup of low-fat yogurt instead will keep them functioning at peak until the last working session of the afternoon.

But you know. And if you want to ensure the success of your meeting, you will have to avoid giving conference attendees too many choices, since the choices they make may be the wrong ones.

You do not give conference-goers the option of choosing the order in which speakers present their talks. Nor do you allow them to decide when sessions are to begin and end or where they are to be held. You control these vital aspects of the conference and feel entirely justified in doing so. You need feel no less justified in taking control of the menu and planning conference meals my way, especially when the results will be so immediately evident and gratifying to all.

Three Days of Breakfast-to-Dinner Conference Eating

All of the brain-powering food principles discussed in this chapter are incorporated in the following menus. You may need to modify them somewhat, depending on your conference budget, the time of year, the location of your meeting, and other variables. Nevertheless, they should serve as useful guidelines to better conference eating and a better experience for all involved.

I know, because my husband and I recently organized a conference on the subject of obesity, sponsored by the New York Academy of Sciences. Several months prior to the meeting, I consulted the individual in charge of menu planning for conferences at the New York hotel where the meeting was to take place. I expressed my desire to have low-fat, alcohol-free lunches, especially since speakers would follow one another at twenty-minute intervals from early morning to late afternoon, and we could not risk an inattentive audience. The caterer was extremely cooperative. The meeting was lively, stimulating, and there was a very high degree of participation in the talks and discussions. In part, this was due to the excellence of the speakers, but credit must be given as well to the mind- and mood-enhancing meals.

Conference Breakfasts

MENU #1
4–6 ounces orange or grapefruit juice
Omelet made from 1 whole egg, 2 egg whites, and mushrooms
2 slices whole-wheat toast
Low-fat milk
Coffee, tea, or decaffeinated beverage as desired

MENU #2
1/2 cantaloupe
2 small or 1 large waffle, topped with a mixture of cottage cheese
   and vanilla yogurt and sprinkled with fresh blueberries, unsweetened granola, and wheat germ
Low-fat milk
Coffee, tea, or decaffeinated beverage as desired

MENU #3
6 ounces orange or cranberry juice
2 crepes, rolled around a mixture of farmer's cheese, raisins, and
   crushed pineapple and topped with lemon-flavored yogurt
Coffee, tea, or decaffeinated beverage as desired

Conference Coffee Breaks, A.M.

Serve a selection of:

Fruit juices
Muffins
Fresh fruits
Coffee and tea (regular and decaffeinated)

Conference Lunches

MENU #1*
1 cup gazpacho Andaluz
3/4 cup salad Niçoise, made with chunks of tuna, whole blanched
string beans, and sliced fresh mushrooms on a bed of lettuce;
garnished with tomato wedges, sliced fresh yellow squash,
blanched broccoli buds, and one sliced new potato
1 tablespoon Dijon vinaigrette dressing
1 whole-wheat and pumpernickel raisin roll
1½ cups sliced fresh fruit in season
Coffee, tea, or decaffeinated beverage as desired

MENU #2*
1 cup cold consommé Madrilene
5 ounces sliced cold breast of chicken on a bed of lettuce
1 cup tortellini salad with pesto dressing, garnished with blanched
broccoli and cauliflower buds, sliced fresh zucchini, and cherry
tomatoes
1 whole-wheat and pumpernickel raisin roll
1 cup raspberry sorbet
Coffee, tea, or decaffeinated beverage as desired

MENU #3
1 cup beef vegetable soup
4 ounces thinly sliced beef with mustard-horseradish sauce
3/4 cup oven-roasted potatoes
½ cup fresh asparagus
½ cup blanched carrots
1 cup fresh fruit cup

*Contributed by the New York Hilton at Rockefeller Center, Harold E. Smith,
Assistant Banquet Manager

Conference Coffee Breaks, P.M.

Serve a selection of:

Frozen yogurt in cups
Trail mix (made with dried fruit, coconut, nuts)
Fresh fruit such as pineapple, strawberries, melon
Coffee, tea (caffeinated and caffeine-free), fruit juices, mineral
  water

or

Barbecued chicken chunks, smoked oysters, boiled shrimp
Raw vegetable crudités with yogurt dip
Zucchini bread, cranberry bread
Popcorn and no-salt pretzels
Coffee, tea (caffeinated and caffeine-free), fruit juices, mineral
  water

Conference Dinners

MENU #1
3/4 cup marinated artichokes
6 ounces poached salmon with mustard dill sauce
4–5 spears steamed broccoli
4 tiny new potatoes
3″ whole-wheat pita bread, toasted
Meringue shell filled with 3/4 cup fresh raspberries

MENU #2
1 cup tomato-clam broth
5 ounces veal marsala
1 cup spinach and mushroom salad
3/4 cup steamed baby carrots with fresh parsley
3/4 cup gnocchi
3 sesame breadsticks
1 medium poached pear filled with 1/2 cup pear sorbet

MENU #3 (reception or buffet)

Choose some or all of the following:

Crudités with cottage cheese or yogurt-based dip
Beef, chicken, and seafood kabobs
Smoked salmon, smoked oysters, smoked duck
Boiled shrimp
Marinated herring, marinated mussels
Marinated mushrooms, marinated artichokes
Miniature tortillas filled with diced chicken
Steamed Chinese dumplings
Blintzes filled with ricotta cheese and topped with caviar
Fresh fruit melange
Fruit kabobs, made with strawberries, pineapple, melon balls

11. How to Eat to Beat Your Inner Clock

A year or so ago I had a client who was attending evening classes to earn a degree in labor relations. Since this attractive young woman worked from nine to five during the day to support herself, she had to do most of her studying on weekends and late at night after classes. She came to me because she had begun to gain weight at an alarming rate. "Could it be all the midnight snacking?" she wondered.

I asked her why she thought she had to eat so much while she studied. Her answer: She needed the energy to stay awake and continue working.

She was in error in believing that she required many extra calories to use her brain into the wee hours. It takes remarkably little food energy to read a book, take notes, and even type a manuscript. But her response alerted me to the fact that she could use my help in another area: maintaining enough brain power and mental energy to think smart during the hours when she normally would be asleep.

I could teach her how to eat to beat the clock. And I can teach you, too!

Loads of extra calories supplied by foods chosen at random won't do it. Determining how you *feel* about your work and then keying foods to your mood is the answer.

For more and more people in our busy society—students and professionals, creative types, business executives, and many others—the traditional eight-hour workday just is not long enough for all the brainwork that needs to be done. Perhaps you are one of them.

Obviously, you can't add more hours to your day. But you can learn special food strategies that will help you use your mind more productively for longer stretches of time—all through the night, if necessary.

Sleep—How Long to Fight It and Why

The writer who must stay up late to meet a deadline, the student who must burn the midnight oil in order to absorb and process reams of information for an exam on the following day, the business person who must remain mentally alert and accurate until dawn to complete a detailed report—for all of them and everyone else who must work smart well past normal bedtime, sleep is the enemy. And it *can* be conquered.

But before I tell you how to use food to face down your body's need for sleep and thus be mentally energetic and efficient for hours longer than you ever thought you could, I must caution you that the techniques you are about to learn are not meant to be used day after day—or night after night.

Even the greatest physical athlete eventually encounters limits to his or her endurance. As a mental competitor, you must realize that you, too, have your limits. Limits vary from person to person, and I cannot predict how long or how hard you will be able to drive yourself before you bump into your own personal limit of mental endurance. But once you reach it, no food strategy will compensate for the brain drain that comes of too many hours of work and too few of rest. At that point, nothing but sleep will refresh and renew your mind so that it can function at peak capacity again.

After one, or at most two, sleepless nights, special eating techniques lose their capability to maintain brain power, and when that happens, only rest will restore top mental form. With that caveat in mind, let's take a closer look at how you can use food to work smarter at least once around the clock without a break.

Obligated or Motivated?
Your Mood Makes a Difference

There actually are two very different food programs that you can use to make your brain function efficiently all through the night. The one you go with should depend on the attitude with which you approach your work, on whether you are feeling obligated or excited.

For example, when you are under intense pressure to complete a job or project on schedule and recognize that the only way to accomplish what must be done is to work through the night, you are feeling obligated. Many students (including the young woman completing her studies in labor relations) and *everyone* rushing to meet a deadline belongs in the obligated category and should follow the food guidelines designed to sustain mental alertness and energy all through the night. The mother or father of a sick or fretting young child, many doctors, and others whose profession requires that they be on call at all hours sometimes belong in the obligated worker category.

Follow the food program for the obligated night worker if, given the choice, you'd rather be in your bed asleep instead of working.

But if you would rather keep on working than knock off for the day and get some rest and relaxation, if you feel compelled to push on not by outside pressure but because you have seized on a concept or theme and simply cannot let go until it has been explored fully, then you obviously are in a highly motivated state. And when that is the case, you will be better able to harness all the mental energy that drives you by following the food program I have developed for the motivated late-night worker.

Remember, every time you settle down for an all-night mental marathon, you will be laboring under one of these two very different states of mind. You will toil until dawn either to meet a deadline or stay on schedule, or you will be spurred on by the challenge of wrestling with a problem and the lure of finding a solution.

State of mind is the single most important factor in determining what, when, and how much to eat to maximize brain power during the hours you normally would be asleep. Before you choose one of the food strategies that follow, decide how you feel about the hours of labor ahead. You'll know. To reiterate, if you'd rather be sleeping, you are in an obligated state. If the work turns you on, you're motivated.

Food Strategies for the Obligated Night Worker

The young woman student mentioned at the beginning of this chapter, who had to study late at night to complete work on her degree, definitely was an obligated worker.

I asked her at our first session whether she had noticed any relation between what she snacked on and how much she was able to accomplish in an evening. She thought for a moment and then remembered the snack she had eaten just the night before: "Two cans of cranberry sauce—the jellied kind, left over from Thanksgiving. It was the only food in the house, so

I dumped some in a bowl and ate it. Twenty minutes later I fell asleep at the kitchen table. Could the cranberry sauce have anything to do with drifting off like that?''

Of course, it did. And you, the reader, can probably guess why. Cranberry sauce is about 50 percent sugar; its very high carbohydrate content was enough to elevate brain serotonin production to the point of causing almost instant sleep.

If my client had eaten the cranberry sauce at noon, it would have decreased her mental energy and motivation and muddled her mind enough to dull her ability to absorb and process information. If she had eaten it at dinner, it would have slowed her thought processes even more; no doubt it would have made her feel drowsy enough to turn in early for the night. But eating it, as she did, at eleven at night, when her mind and body were wound down and prepared for sleep, was tantamount to taking a powerful sleeping pill.

Remember, your mind is normally at its keenest and most alert in the first few hours after you awaken in the morning. And because all your biological rhythms are in high gear at that time, your mind is also least vulnerable to the effects of food. But as the day wears on and your biological rhythms progress through the slow, winding-down process that eventually readies you for sleep, the food you eat becomes more and more important in determining mental energy and mood.

When you need to work late and work smart, you must fight the strong tendency of your body to follow its normal twenty-four-hour sleep/wake cycle, a cycle which dictates that as night approaches, body temperature will drop, metabolism will slow, production of some hormones will decrease while that of others increases dramatically . . . and feelings of hunger will dwindle down to practically nothing.

How do you fight this tendency to go to sleep? By using food to fool your body into delaying some of its preparations for rest and to prevent it from manufacturing substances such as serotonin, which invite sleepiness.

Eating for a Successful Late-Night Work Marathon

Here's how to eat for a successful late-night work marathon.

Have dinner as late as possible—at nine or nine-thirty in the evening, if you can wait that long. The rationale: A delayed evening meal will force your body to work hard at digestion much later in the day than is usual. Since digestion temporarily increases metabolism, your system will have to continue what are normally daytime metabolic processes for a few hours longer.

If you think delaying dinner for such a long time will leave you too hungry to function efficiently earlier in the evening, plan ahead by rescheduling and modifying all of your meals that day. Have the equivalent of half your usual lunch at noon, for example, then eat the other half, or a snack, at five or five-thirty in the afternoon. This late half-lunch or snack will get you through until dinner at nine.

Make sure that your delayed dinner is a real meal.

- It should include between four and six ounces of protein, one or two cups of vegetables (leafy green and bright-colored), and a small serving—one cup or less—of carbohydrate, such as rice or potatoes. For dessert, have an apple, orange, banana, berries, or other fruit.
- Your delayed dinner should be low in fat. That means no butter or margarine on bread, vegetables, rice, or potato, and no more than a teaspoon of oil on your salad. (Low-calorie, oil-free dressing would be better still.)
- Begin your meal with protein. It will help block the production of sleep-inducing serotonin. Don't start to eat carbohydrates until you have finished all of the protein.
- The protein component of your meal should be fish, other seafood, poultry, veal, or lean beef (grilled or roasted and trimmed of all visible fat). Remember that while meats

such as pork, ham, and lamb, and dairy products, such as hard cheese, are also protein foods, they are very high in fat, thus contributing to mental slowdown.

If you normally drink caffeinated beverages, drink a cup of coffee or tea at the conclusion of your delayed dinner.
If you know earlier in the day that you will be working late that night, you can increase the brain-stimulating effects of caffeine after dinner by drinking much less coffee or tea than usual (or none at all) after your first cup at breakfast. When you avoid caffeine for many hours, caffeine levels in your system will drop well below what is normal for you, and you will experience greater sensitivity to this substance when you resume consumption after dinner.

Once you have started to work, take a food break every two or three hours or so. The reason for putting more food into your system at frequent intervals is *not* to fulfill a need for calories. (After all, you will be engaging in mental, not physical labor, and even if your job for the night is to watch over a sick child or to tend patients in a hospital emergency room, your delayed dinner will have supplied you with enough food energy to see you through.) Rather, small frequent snacks will force your body to maintain a higher metabolic rate and thus prevent your system from shutting down to normal nocturnal levels, thereby turning you off mentally. It's a way of using food to interrupt and prolong the waking part of your sleep/wake cycle.

What kind of food should you eat?

- Low-fat proteins such as tuna and other canned fish, cold, lean meat, poached eggs, cottage cheese, and low-fat yogurt are best because of their capacity to stimulate production of the alertness chemicals.
- Next best are the nonstarchy vegetables and fruits such as carrots, celery, red and green peppers, and broccoli, as well as apples, oranges, bananas, berries, peaches, plums,

and even dried fruits such as raisins, dates, figs, and dried apricots. All will help keep your metabolic processes up closer to daytime levels without increasing serotonin production.

- Soybean snacks, peanuts, and other nuts contain carbohydrates, but because they are also high in protein, which helps prevent the brain from making serotonin, they won't cause late-night mental capabilities to take a nose dive. (However, keep in mind that because nuts are so high in calories, enough of them *will* add pounds to your weight.)
- *Do not eat sweet or starchy foods unaccompanied by protein.* Cookies, candy, ice cream, cake, potato chips, pretzels, bread or toast with or without jam, and all—I repeat, *all*—other sweet or starchy foods will decrease dramatically your ability to stay awake, motivated, and clear-headed.

From time to time during the night you will experience an almost irresistible urge to eat carbohydrates. Be prepared! The craving is your body's way of attempting to trick you into doing what it wants to do: get some sleep. In fact, if you give in to it, you may as well brush your teeth, climb into your pajamas, and kiss your work good-night. You won't be able to function at the peak of your mental powers again until morning.

Assuming that you are not overly sensitive to caffeine, have coffee or tea with every food break. It will help prevent brain blur and keep mental energy and accuracy up where you want them.

Take time off to exercise. Although this is a book about managing your mind and your moods with food, a few words about exercise are in order here.

Physical activity, like the process of digestion, will cause a temporary speed-up in your metabolism and slightly elevate your temperature above normal nocturnal levels. Temperature and metabolism both drop at night, and short, vigorous bouts of activity, which briefly bring them back up to daytime levels, are thus another means of fooling your body into staying awake, further prolonging your ability to work smart into the night.

The question of how much and how often to exercise during a night-long work marathon is a difficult one to answer. Certainly, if you are out of shape and haven't acquired the habit of regular physical activity, you should not try anything strenuous like running twice around the block. However, even if you are relatively unfit, you can still move vigorously enough to get your blood flowing faster, increase your metabolism, and slightly raise your temperature. Try some easy stretching and bending, followed by a few minutes of sit-ups, push-ups, or running in place. Stop when you feel your body becoming warmer and your head beginning to clear. (An exercise bike is especially useful because you can climb on and pedal furiously for about five minutes or until your brain is back in high gear.) Even just getting up from your desk, walking a few times around the room, stretching, and shaking out your hands, arms, and legs will help counter the drop in metabolism and body temperature that promote sleepiness.

Damage Limitation Techniques for the Morning After

You may be surprised at how peppy you feel and how well you function in the morning after a marathon work night. Assuming that you *do* feel energetic in those first early hours of the day, it is because your body's biological rhythms are all on the upswing in the morning, despite your interrupting your sleep/wake cycle the night before. Indeed, many people who stay up all night remark that even if they have time to sleep at six or seven in the morning, they often can't.

Nevertheless, the biological clock that turns you on in the morning even when you have not slept the night before continues ticking as the day progresses. And from about noon on, you will become more and more vulnerable to mind fatigue as your need for sleep reasserts itself.

If you are not to collapse into a quivering mass of sleep-deprived protoplasm, *you must continue to eat protein before carbohydrate* at every meal and snack throughout the day.

And, unless you are one of those people who simply cannot tolerate any caffeine *ever,* you should increase your intake of coffee or tea. But don't take caffeine until you need it. If you are feeling alert and bright of mind and eye, delay your first cup until your lids begin to droop and your mind to blur. This may occur as early as ten o'clock or not until after lunch. When it does, take a double dose to jolt your brain awake again. And from then on, drink enough to keep you going. Do not worry about being hyper. As the day progresses, you will become more and more *hypo,* and will need the extra caffeine to stay on your feet until bedtime.

A Beat-the-Clock Food Plan for the Obligated All-Night Mental Worker

These sample dinner, snack, and morning-after breakfast suggestions will boost your brain power and help you stay alert and motivated from sundown to sunup. They'll work even if your project is a bore, the material difficult, and you long to be rid of it all. However, you *must* give it a chance by following instructions to the letter. It is imperative that you delay dinner for as long as possible and that you snack on schedule in order to keep your stomach and other digestive organs busy and your metabolism elevated. The key to maintaining mental energy all through the night is to make your body work as if it were day.

DINNER
4–5 ounces fish, chicken, veal, or lean beef
1 medium potato or 1 cup rice

1 medium portion salad consisting of assorted raw vegetables such as spinach, tomatoes, cucumbers, raw mushrooms, broccoli, cauliflower

1 cup cooked vegetables such as green beans, squash, or carrots

1 piece fresh fruit such as a banana, orange, or apple or 1 cup strawberries or blueberries or ½ grapefruit or melon

SNACKS

Every three hours, exercise to get your body temperature and metabolism up, then have one item from the following list:

4 ounces cottage cheese

4 ounces low-fat plain, vanilla, or lemon-flavored yogurt

3–4 sardines or 1–2 ounces herring

1–2 ounces cooked chicken, lean roast beef, tuna, or salmon

1 cup beef-vegetable soup

1 cup fish or clam chowder made with tomato stock or milk, not cream

1–2 slices low-fat mozarella cheese

1 ounce feta cheese

1–2 hard-boiled eggs. (Because of their high cholesterol content, you should eat no more than three "visible" eggs per week; do not eat eggs if you have already consumed your quota.)

¾ cup of the following vegetables, raw or cooked, and sliced: carrots, cherry tomatoes, red cabbage, red or green pepper, mushrooms, celery, cucumber, pickles, asparagus, broccoli, cauliflower

1 banana

¾ cup pineapple (if canned, should be packed in its own juice)

1 orange

½ grapefruit

½ melon

¾ cup berries of any kind

1 pear

1 apple

1 peach

1 frozen fruit puree pop, unsweetened

Note: Do not eat grapes on a marathon work night. They are high in glucose, the sugar that promotes tryptophan uptake in the brain and spurs the production of the relaxing chemical, serotonin.

When thirsty, drink water, seltzer, mineral water, or eight ounces of fruit juice; or have a cup of clear vegetable, chicken, or beef soup or broth.

DAY-AFTER BREAKFAST. Because you have been up and working for hours, you may be hungrier for breakfast than usual and the two day-after breakfasts below take that fact into account. Just remember, after an all-nighter, you *must* avoid carbohydrates unless accompanied by protein. Otherwise you will be groggy by three o'clock in the afternoon.

BREAKFAST #1
1 cup strawberries, mixed with
1 cup cottage cheese and sprinkled with
1 tablespoon unsweetened granola, served on
1 slice frozen French toast or waffle
Coffee, tea, or low-fat milk

BREAKFAST #2
4–6 ounces of orange or grapefruit juice
2 poached eggs on
1 English muffin, *very* lightly buttered
Coffee, tea, or low-fat milk

Food Strategies for the Motivated Night Worker

Let's say you are feeling enthusiastic, turned-on, *passionate* about a project, that you are eager to start the job and see it through to completion, instead of wishing it would somehow get done by itself while you are snoozing peacefully in your bed. When that is the case, the food strategies that will help you work smarter all through the night are very different from those I recommend to the less fervent, obligated night worker.

When you are full of zeal and impatient to get going and keep going, you should have little or no problem staying awake. But after a few hours of high-energy mental labor you may begin to feel overexcited, less focused, and less able to deal with the frustration of failing to find immediate, successful solutions to the problems posed by your work.

Among my clients are a number of young men and women who are self-admitted "computer hacks." One of them told me that if I were to go into the computer room on a Monday morning after four or five of them had been working there all weekend, it would look like Halloween: "You'll be wading knee-deep in wrappers from Twinkies, candy bars, vending machine cookies and crackers, cans of soda, Popsicle sticks, and empty crumpled potato chip and pretzel bags."

What does all the trash on the computer room floor say about these super-committed all-night toilers? Think about it a moment, and you will realize that this isn't just any old trash but trash left over after eating *carbohydrate* foods. These computer types, as they work through the night, instinctively obey their bodies' demands for sweets and starches. But in the highly motivated mental state of the computer hack, that demand does not arise from the body's need to slow down and get some sleep. Rather, the carbohydrate craving represents an attempt on the part of the brain to focus and refocus rapidly on frequent ideas and impose some order on churning thought processes.

Throughout this book I have emphasized the calming, relaxing, and frequently soporific effects of carbohydrates. I often have cautioned you against eating sweets or starches when you want to be at your sharpest and most alert. I even have warned you that in many instances eating even a small amount of carbohydrate will trigger the production of enough serotonin to put you to sleep within minutes. These effects have been demonstrated time and again in our lab at M.I.T. and at other scientific research organizations.

But it is also true that in a few special circumstances—as when your brain is working so fast and furiously that it is difficult to sort the important ideas from the ideas that will lead nowhere—carbohydrates will help slow the unproductive spinning of your mind and allow you to zero in on the details of your work.

There is a good neurochemical basis for the enormous craving for carbohydrates sometimes felt by enthusiastic, super-motivated creative people. When you are intensely engaged in original thinking, your brain may be spewing ideas so quickly that it is almost impossible to pin them down. As an artistic friend told me, "Occasionally, when I work on a painting, something takes hold of me, and I can't make my brush move fast enough to keep up with the images in my mind." I have had writer colleagues tell me that at times, when they are in the throes of the creative process, the words come so rapidly that they cannot keep pace, no matter how fast they scribble or type. I have heard essentially the same comments from computer hacks, inventors, and business people.

I call this state "creative overload"—too many ideas flooding the circuits too quickly to be evaluated and processed in an orderly manner. Serotonin will help by slowing the output of rapid, random thoughts, allowing you to organize, structure, and direct them toward creative problem-solving.

When you are hopped up mentally about a project, the following food guidelines will help you deal with creative overload. They'll enable you to control the flood of ideas and make them work better for you.

Plan to have dinner as late as possible. This will keep your stomach "awake" and busy with digestion much later into the evening than usual. And by delaying digestion, a process that requires an expenditure of energy, you will also be prolonging the period before your metabolism dips down to its normal nighttime low. When you want to work hard and work smart all through the night, it is important to keep your metabolism in sync with the high-level activity of your mind.

If you are ordinarily an early eater and foresee hunger problems if you don't start dinner at the usual hour, you can use the strategy I recommended for obligated workers in the same predicament: Plan ahead. Eat only half of your usual lunch at midday and save the other half to eat as a snack at five o'clock. This late-afternoon mini-meal should tide you over until you sit down to your delayed dinner at eight-thirty or nine.

Don't skimp on your late dinner. It should include all the components of a full meal, similar to what is suggested for your counterpart, the obligated worker: Begin with four to six ounces of protein. Have a salad or serving of leafy green vegetables and a serving of a bright-colored vegetable. You should also have a cup or less of a starchy food such as rice or potatoes. (Or, if you prefer, omit the starch and eat two slices of bread, unbuttered.) Dessert should be fruit—any kind, so long as it is not sweetened with sugar, served in a heavy, sugary syrup, or covered with whipped cream. (For more details on what to eat for dinner before you settle down to a night of creative work, turn back to page 192 and reread the bulleted material.)

Do not conclude your delayed meal with coffee or tea or drink any beverages containing caffeine (including cola drinks and cocoa) after dinner. In fact, you should avoid caffeinated drinks entirely during your long night of mental labor unless, or until, you begin to feel your brain running out of go-power. In your highly motivated, super-enthusiastic mental state, the additional stimulation that caffeine will provide is not only unnecessary, it might push you over the dividing line between feeling hyper-alert and efficient and being too jangled to apply your mind effectively.

You are excused from following this important no-caffeine-after-dinner rule if you are a coffee or tea addict accustomed to very high levels of caffeine in your body at all times. For you, even temporary withdrawal may result in a mental crash that will hinder your ability to perform.

Once every two or three hours—or whenever the thoughts begin to fly in and out of your head too rapidly to process and apply to the problems at hand—take a carbohydrate snack break.

Within a very short while after eating a sweet or starchy food, the amino acid tryptophan will enter your brain in amounts sufficient to produce more serotonin. Serotonin, in turn, will make you feel more composed, less distractible. Your state of mind will literally go from unfocused to focused in ten to fifteen minutes!

The best carbohydrate foods to eat when you are working through the night are those that contain little or no fat, so they will be digested quickly and rapidly exert their calming, focusing effect on your mind.

When it's time for a carbohydrate break, choose from the snacks below. They are listed in order from most desirable— that is, lowest in fat, easiest to digest, and quickest-acting—to somewhat desirable. In a pinch, even the snack foods at the very bottom of the list will be enormously effective in calming hyperactive thought processes, enabling you to refocus and reapply yourself to your work.

- Regular—*not* dietetic or sugar-free—soft drinks, especially those that are caffeine-free. (Of course, when you feel the need for a caffeine pickup, then one of the caffeinated brands would be the drink of choice.) I have ranked soft drinks up at the very top of the list because they go down quickly—no need even to chew!—and are digested more easily and rapidly than solid foods. In fact, results are almost instant.
- Low-fat candies, such as gumdrops, jelly beans, licorice sticks, and marshmallows. These, too, are pure sugar, but

I've put them in second place because they require some chewing and must spend a few more moments being digested in the stomach before they are ready to travel through the blood as glucose, ultimately spurring the production of serotonin.

- Dry cereal (presweetened for an extra shot of sugar), popcorn, Cracker Jacks, and low- or no-salt pretzels. These foods require a bit more in the way of digestion than those listed above, and thus lag a few moments behind in triggering serotonin production.
- Packaged pastries and other sweet carbohydrates, such as Twinkies, chocolate cupcakes, cookies (plain and cream-filled), nougat or caramel candy bars, and fudge-type candies. All of these contain more fat than the foods in the first three categories and therefore should be considered last-resort calmers, since they take longer to work.

Exercise from time to time throughout the night. If your mind is racing, you won't need bouts of physical activity to stay awake. Nevertheless, your biological clock dictates that your body cool somewhat during the hours you would normally be asleep. When you are intent on your work—whether you are sitting at a desk or in front of a word processor, or even standing before an easel—you are not moving around or using your muscles to any significant degree. This relative immobility allows the cool-down process to proceed. Thus, what is happening in your brain is incompatible with the state of your body: The first is heated and active, the latter is cooled and inert. (Brain-body incompatibility may be especially pronounced in the computer hack who works in a room that is climate-controlled to protect the hardware.)

Exercise is important, then, because it will increase your metabolism, warm your body, and bring it into synchrony with your brain.

It takes very little in the way of physical activity to speed up your metabolism enough to warm up your body: Every hour or so, simply get up and stretch your back, arm, and leg muscles, then do a few minutes of sit-ups or push-ups or jog in place. If you are not that ambitious, stretching and then pacing around the room for five minutes will do it. So will walking briskly up and down a flight of stairs.

Morning-After Rise-and-Shine Strategies

It would be ideal if you could manage a couple of hours of sleep before greeting the day, especially if you have an exam or presentation coming up in the morning. But even if you had the time, you might find it difficult to fall asleep, since your biological rhythms are now on the early-morning upswing.

Nevertheless, the mountainous mental high you have been on all night will soon diminish to a tiny molehill, and after the peak in your biological rhythms, you will no longer be able to count on sheer motivation and enthusiasm to sustain brain power.

What you need now is a fresh infusion of tyrosine, the amino acid that stimulates production of the alertness chemicals, dopamine and norepinephrine. The source of tyrosine is, of course, protein. To stay as alert as possible for as long as possible, your first meal of the day—and every meal and snack thereafter until you are back on a normal sleep schedule— *must* be high in protein.

Poached eggs, low-fat cottage cheese, chicken, tuna, yogurt, lean hamburger, and even lean roast beef are all good breakfast choices for the morning after a work binge. The fact that these foods are low in fat is almost as important as their high protein content, since in your sleep-deprived state, you will be especially vulnerable to the grogginess and lethargy associated with high-fat eating.

As for caffeine, don't drink coffee or tea first thing in the morning if you don't need it. Wait until you begin to feel brain-drained and muddled. Then have a cup or two of your favorite beverage to jolt your mind back to a normal state of alertness.

A Beat-the-Clock Food Plan for the Motivated All-Night Mental Laborer

Computer scientists, creative writers and artists, scientists, entrepreneurs, and a host of others who often are too absorbed in their work to leave some of it undone until morning have had great success with the following dinner, snack, and morning-after breakfast menus. Keep in mind that dinner must be eaten as late in the evening as possible and that, as a motivated worker whose mind is churning with so many ideas it may be difficult to concentrate fully on the details of a project, it is imperative that you avoid protein snacks and caffeine until you are finished for the night.

DINNER (Delay until 8:30 or 9:00 P.M., if you can.)

5 ounces fish, chicken, veal, or lean beef, roasted or grilled
1 medium baked potato
1/2 cup raw vegetables such as red cabbage, red or green pepper, or broccoli
1/2–3/4 cup cooked vegetables such as string beans, yellow squash, snow peas, spinach
1 cup fresh fruit salad

SNACKS

Approximately every two hours, exercise, then have one of the following snacks. This is but a *very* general guideline, however, since your mental processes will have their own schedule. For example, in the early part of your all-night work marathon, you may become distracted or feel your thoughts begin to "spin" as often as every thirty or forty-five minutes. Don't wait the full two hours for a carbohydrate snack; have something as soon as you are aware of the developing problem. Later on, when you are settled into a work groove, you may need to snack only once every three or four hours.

All of the following snacks are listed in 100-calorie amounts. Try not to exceed that dosage, since the calories *will* add up.

1 can soda
1 1-ounce Tootsie roll
4 small wrapped caramel candies
8 large jelly beans
20 pieces candy corn
8 graham crackers
1¼ cups Cheerios
1 cup Corn Chex
⅔ cup Wheat Chex
1 ounce pretzels, low-salt

DAY-AFTER BREAKFAST. After an all-night work session, you will probably be hungrier than usual, thus the menus that follow are planned to satisfy a larger than normal breakfast appetite. Although this meal *must* be high in protein, there is no reason why it should be limited to traditional breakfast fare.

BREAKFAST MENU #1
½ grapefruit
3 ounces of tuna or chicken, mixed with no more than
½ tablespoon mayonnaise or salad dressing
3″ pita bread
Coffee, tea, or low-fat milk

BREAKFAST MENU #2
2 slices *very lean* ham on
2 slices whole-wheat toast, topped with
1 slice melted low-fat cheese,
4–5 ounces orange or grapefruit juice
Coffee, tea, or low-fat milk

12. Travelers' Advisory: Anti–Jet Lag Tactics for Better Business and Pleasure Trips

The brain and body fatigue caused by jet lag are nuisance enough when you are traveling for pleasure. But when work is the reason for a journey, the consequences can be serious indeed.

One of my clients, a top sales representative for a large, high-tech electronics firm, came to me soon after returning from a business trip to France. He had been scheduled to make an important presentation to potential customers the morning after his arrival in Paris. The meeting was set for ten o'clock, a reasonable hour, but for my client, still functioning on Boston time, it was as though he had been roused from bed at four in the morning to make a major sales pitch.

He is an assertive, articulate man who normally speaks with great ease, eloquence, and conviction—but not at the Paris meeting. He said, "I felt as if I were underwater. Even though I knew what I wanted to say and how I wanted to say it, my thoughts had to float up from the depths before I could turn

them into words. It was one of the most important presentations of my career, and my mind was so slowed-down, I
almost struck out."

My advice to him—and to you whenever you plan to travel
through several time zones—is to be aware in advance that
your brain and body will not immediately function up to their
"home" performance level. Give yourself time to adjust.
Arrange your itinerary so that there is a buffer day between
your arrival and any demanding activity, whether business or
pleasure.

Just as important, use anti–jet lag food strategies that will
speed the adjustment.

West-to-East Eating Schedule

Traveling from west to east—for example, from California
to New York or from New York to Brussels or Rome—is more
difficult in terms of jet lag than going in the opposite direction.
(An explanation follows later in this chapter.) Yet I have met
many European colleagues and friends who are amazed at the
way Americans seem to adapt so quickly to eating and sleeping in time zones that are six or eight hours ahead of their
home zones. The Europeans are impressed by the fact that
most of us refuse to take it easy on arrival and instead plunge
immediately into business and recreational activities.

Around the world, we're still seen as go-getters, because
that is what so many of us are. I suspect that although we
touch down in a new time zone as out of sync with food and
sleep needs as travelers from other lands, we are just too
determined to make the best use of our time to let these
"minor" problems interfere. Unfortunately, jet lag does interfere, as so many of even my most dynamic clients have
testified.

The sheer determination to keep moving won't hasten the
adjustment from jet-lagged brain functioning to maximum

mental alertness and energy. But the special west-to-east food guidelines I have developed will.

Here's what to do.

Before You Leave

Switch into the eating and sleeping schedule of your destination time zone as soon as possible. It won't be practical to begin making adjustments the day before you leave, but you will certainly be able to start adapting a few hours before your departure, thus giving yourself a head start in resetting your biological clock.

Let's assume that you are going to Europe and that your plane is scheduled to take off in the evening, as so many eastbound transatlantic flights do.

On the day of your flight, eat a normal breakfast, consisting of the same amount and kind of food that you usually have in the morning.

At lunch, have a large, "dinnerlike" meal, similar in quantity and variety of foods to what you ordinarily eat in the evening (i.e., a four- to six-ounce serving of fish, chicken, or meat; a salad; some vegetables, including a starchy vegetable such as rice or a potato; and dessert, if you normally finish dinner with a sweet).

Drink your last cup of coffee or tea for the day at lunchtime. Avoid *all* caffeinated beverages for the next several hours. (If you are not a caffeine freak and can function fairly well without it, it would be even better if you stopped drinking coffee or tea still earlier in the day, after breakfast.)

If you want something to eat at midafternoon, make it a carbohydrate snack. Good choices: a bagel, an English muffin, a bran or corn muffin, crackers, or cookies. Eat no protein for the time being.

Before you board your plane, have a dinner composed of high-carbohydrate foods such as pasta or a noodle or rice dish.

If your flight leaves at about the time you would ordinarily have your evening meal, eat early, before takeoff. The idea is to fill up with enough carbohydrate food to make you feel pleasantly full and to induce your brain to make more serotonin, the calming chemical. I want you to be well-fed and relaxed when you board the plane—well-fed enough not to need to eat dinner on the aircraft and relaxed enough to sleep through most of the flight.

Special to
Midwesterners and Westerners

If you must leave early in the day to connect with a transatlantic flight from the East Coast, eat the airline lunch served on your connecting flight. Try to skip coffee or tea at lunchtime. (If you must have a cup of your favorite caffeinated beverage then, make it your last one of the day.) Your afternoon snack, if you have one, should consist of carbohydrate foods only. (If you will be in flight at snack time, take gumdrops, jelly beans, caramels, licorice, or crackers with you. Many airlines serve just a package of nuts at midafternoon.) While waiting for your plane to Europe, have a quick high-carbohydrate dinner at the airport restaurant. Once again, the idea is to avoid eating dinner on the plane. I want you to be comfortably full of carbohydrates when you board so that you will be more likely to sleep most of the time you are airborne.

On the Plane

Do not eat on the plane. Instead, sleep as much as you can. Getting to sleep early and staying asleep for most of your flight is extremely important when your goal is to adjust quickly to the food and sleep schedules of your destination time zone in the east. If wine makes you feel drowsy, have a glass or two when they wheel the drinks cart down the aisle. Then ask for a blanket (pressurized cabins can be chilly) and eyeshades (if light tends to keep you awake). Tell flight attendants not to wake you if you are asleep when dinner is served.

If you ordinarily have trouble getting to sleep on a plane or if you will be en route many hours before your usual bedtime, you might even want to consider using a mild sleeping pill. There are new drugs that will help you fall asleep almost instantly but have such short-term effects (they work for only four or five hours) that you won't be groggy when you touch down. Tell your physician your reason for wanting one. If he or she agrees that it is a good idea, take one of these pills soon after you board your plane.

If your destination is Western Europe (as opposed to points farther east or south), ask to be awakened for breakfast. On European flights, this meal is served approximately ninety minutes before landing—somewhere between midnight and 3 A.M. in your home time zone. Force yourself to have at least juice and coffee.

A word of caution: Assuming you are hungry enough, have eggs if they are served, but go easy on carbohydrate foods such as rolls, toast, croissants, etc. Because your body is still functioning on its home zone schedule—where it is still so early in the morning that you ordinarily would be sleeping—a high-carbohydrate breakfast will promote serotonin production and make you feel even drowsier when you arrive. Juice, however, is okay.

If you are flying past Western Europe (to, say, Israel or Hungary), tell flight attendants to let you sleep through breakfast as well as dinner. When you awaken, ask for coffee or tea. They are almost always available up to the time the cabin crew closes the galley, just before landing.

Once You Have Landed

Once you have arrived at your destination, eat according to the normal pattern in your new time zone. Mealtimes may roll around well before you have worked up an appetite, and you may not be hungry on schedule. Eat anyway. It will help your brain and your body adjust more quickly and thus enable you to function better sooner.

What you eat is as important as when you eat. The wrong food at the wrong time may result in grogginess and fatigue just when you want to be your most mentally energetic and alert. Conversely, the wrong food can reinforce your body's inclination to become more and more awake and less likely to settle into sleep when it is bedtime in your destination time zone.

Which Foods When

The basic anti–jet lag food rule when you travel from west to east is simple:

- Breakfast and lunch should be high in protein.
- Dinner and any snacks eaten thereafter should consist mainly of carbohydrates.

Protein eaten early in the day will help keep you mentally wide awake, even though your internal clock, still set on home zone time, tells you it's time to sleep. Carbohydrates eaten late in the day will help you feel relaxed and somewhat slowed down at a time when, if you were home, you would just be getting into mental and physical high gear.

BREAKFASTS. Finding a proper west-to-east anti–jet lag breakfast may pose a problem or two. To counter your body's desire to continue sleeping, the first meal of the day should supply plenty of protein. However, the typical morning meal in many Western European countries is very low in protein (I am thinking now of a croissant with jam and coffee, which often passes for breakfast in France). Or the breakfast protein is too high in fat (as in Holland, for example, where hard cheese and cold meats are often served in the morning). Too much fat, of course, will dull your mind and exaggerate feelings of fatigue.

Nevertheless, even when these problems exist, you do have options:

- You can pay extra at your hotel, and order eggs or yogurt if they are on the menu.
- Or you can buy yogurt and low-fat soft cheese, such as cottage cheese, to eat in your room. (Stow it in the refrigerator with which, as noted, almost all European hotel rooms are equipped.)

You will find that buying food as a traveler in Europe, where most hotels are situated in the middle of a city or small town, is often easier than here, where many hotels are surrounded by major highways and acres of parking lots that must be negotiated to reach a grocery store or supermarket. You may also be surprised to discover that in Europe, major department stores almost always have an entire floor stocked with food, including dairy products and fresh produce!

Or you can simply eat very little of the high-carbohydrate and/or high-fat meal served at your hotel. It will be easier to avoid mental sluggishness if you nibble lightly at a single roll or a small piece of hard cheese than if you eat these same foods in meal-size amounts.

Also, if you can tolerate caffeine at all, first thing in the morning is the time for a cup or two of coffee or tea. The extra stimulation caffeine provides can make all the difference between having that sleeping-with-your-eyes-open feeling for the first part of the day and functioning more or less normally.

A.M. EXERCISE EXTRA! Try to do something moderately strenuous for a few minutes after you get out of bed. A few push-ups or sit-ups or some jogging in place will raise your body temperature enough from its home time zone low—remember, if you were at home, you would still be sleeping—to nudge your biological clock forward to correspond more closely to the sleep-wake cycle of the new time zone.

But do *not* exercise after midafternoon. When the goal is to overcome west-to-east jet lag, you must encourage your body to wind down as the day progresses. Physical activity late in the day—when, if you were at home, you would just be hitting your mental and physical stride—will only prolong the period of adjustment.

LUNCHES. No matter where in the world you are, you will have a greater choice of foods at midday than you did in the morning, and it should be easy to find the high-protein meals that will keep you mentally "up" for the next few hours.

Begin lunch with a low-fat source of protein such as fish, other seafood, poultry, veal or beef (trimmed of all fat), or a low-fat cheese or other dairy product. In selecting proteins that are low in fat, you will be protecting yourself against the inevitable grogginess that follows a highly caloric meal.

Be sure to avoid other sources of fat as well! No butter, heavy sauces, or creamed soups. Use salad dressing sparingly, and don't eat more than a bite or two of cheese if it is one of the high-fat varieties, such as goat cheese or Brie.

Keep carbohydrate intake low. One roll, a medium potato, or one cup of rice or noodles would be safe—provided, of course, that you don't eat carbohydrate before the protein component of your meal.

Drink no wine at lunch unless you plan on following it with a nap. Wine will prolong jet lag.

Finish lunch with coffee or tea. It will help keep your mind from fogging up later on.

DINNERS. If you are several time zones east of your home zone, you may have little interest in breakfast or lunch the first couple of days after you arrive. That is because you will be eating these meals when you would normally be sleeping, and your biological clock says it is not yet time to eat.

Dinner, though, is a different matter. If you are in Western Europe, for example, you will be sitting down to this meal at a time that corresponds roughly to midday in your home zone, when your biological clock is telling you to fill up. Moreover, after hours of feeling mentally muddled and physically fatigued, you will probably, finally, be fully awake.

As I mentioned earlier, the basic anti–jet lag rule for west-to-east travelers is to keep protein low and carbohydrates high at dinner. If you don't—if, for instance, you eat more than four ounces of fish, other seafood, poultry, red meat, or cheese—the alertness chemicals that can flood out from your brain after protein is ingested may keep you tossing and turning in your bed long after most people in the new time zone are soundly sleeping.

Staying awake late and consequently awakening late the next morning may not pose major problems if you are on vacation and simply want to relax and take it easy. But when you travel for business or professional reasons and fail to make a quick mental and physical adjustment, the consequences can be unfortunate for your firm—and perhaps your career.

In any case, I urge you to plan dinner as a prelude to sleep, at least for the first two or three days in the new time zone. That means, in addition to keeping protein intake low, *starting your meal with a carbohydrate food*. (Remember, if you start with protein, serotonin production will be blocked.)

Begin your meal, then, with bread, breadsticks or rolls, an appetizer course of pasta, puff pastry, or a crepe filled with vegetables.

Order a starch—pasta, noodles, rice, or potato—as part of your main course, and eat it before you begin on the protein.

Have no more than four ounces of protein. Less would be

better. One way to be sure you won't exceed the four-ounce limit is to order a dish—for example, a casserole or crepe—in which fish, another seafood, poultry, or meat is only one of many ingredients. Another way to keep protein intake low is to order an appetizer (because it's small) in place of an entrée. An appetizer-size portion of smoked salmon or duck, oysters, or marinated mussels, for example, would supply you with just about the right amount of good, low-fat protein.

Have a glass or two of wine with dinner. Alcohol may help make you sleepy.

Order dessert unless you are watching your waistline. The additional carbohydrate will help finish the job that began with the high-carbohydrate appetizer. (Keep in mind that fruit—unless it is served in syrup, glazed, or otherwise sugared—will have no sleep-inducing effect.)

If you want to linger on at your table with coffee or tea, specify the decaffeinated kind.

BEDTIME SNACKS. Reinforce the effects of your high-carbohydrate dinner with a sweet snack about an hour before you plan to settle in to sleep. Any sweet cookie, cake, or candy will do.

Still feeling too active and "up" to drift off to sleep? A leisurely drink will help you unwind the rest of the way. Some brandy or cognac (buy a tiny bottle on the airplane) will be a delicious accompaniment to your sweet snack and should push you over the edge of wakefulness into slumber. But do not overdo alcohol. Too much actually can *interfere* with sleep!

If you should drift off only to awaken two or three hours later, bright-eyed and ready to take on the new day—except that it is still the middle of the night in your new time zone—have another sweet snack. It will enable you to get a few more hours of slumber.

My west-to-east food guidelines won't do away completely with jet lag, but they will lessen its effect. And if you begin early enough—before you board the aircraft, if possible—I can promise that you will feel more fully awake and mentally energetic from the moment you touch down than if you do what comes naturally and maintain your home zone eating and sleeping patterns into your destination time zone.

How long should you follow the anti–jet lag food plan? Stay with it for the first two days after your arrival. If you still have that blurred, half hung-over feeling in the morning of day three, continue the food plan throughout the third day.

One more thing: You needn't wait until your next trip to Europe to benefit from these west-to-east food guidelines. They will be equally helpful in allaying jet lag whenever you travel in an easterly direction. Californians, for example, will find the guidelines invaluable when they visit New York. And business people who have spent enough time in the Far East to adapt to Oriental food and sleep schedules can use the eating plan to readjust on their return home to the States.

East-to-West Eating Schedule

A series of fascinating studies designed to determine what our natural sleep/wake cycle would be if we were guided only by our own biological rhythms and not influenced by externals (such as clocks, as well as sunrises and sunsets) indicates that there is a tendency to extend each day by going to sleep an hour or so later every night.

This may explain why so many world travelers have less trouble with jet lag when they fly in a *westerly* direction, as opposed to going toward the east. As we have just seen, in adjusting to a time zone that is east of your home zone, you must make an effort to get to sleep *earlier* for the first couple of nights after you arrive. Going to sleep hours before normal bedtime feels less comfortable—because it is contrary to biological rhythms—than going to sleep later, which is what you must train yourself to do when you travel across time zones to the west.

Of course, skipping westward across many time zones, as when you travel from the East Coast to Hawaii or from the West Coast to Japan or Hong Kong, will nevertheless leave you jet lagged and cause a temporary but marked decrease in mental sharpness. Even returning home to the United States from a stay in Europe—if you became completely adjusted to European food and sleep schedules—will leave you feeling brain drained and muddled until you readjust.

So, although east-to-west jet lag may not be quite as difficult to deal with, you will still need all the help you can get if you are to regain your home zone brain power quickly and function at peak soon after an east-to-west flight.

Eating the right food, at the right time, is the key.

Before You Leave

These east-to-west anti–jet lag strategies are all designed to reset your biological clock *back* by a few hours, since in time zones to the west, you will be doing everything—waking, eating, going to bed—*later* than in your home zone.

Thus, on the morning of your westward journey, sleep as late as possible to enable yourself to stay awake well past your normal bedtime that night.

Eat a small breakfast—no more than a piece of toast or a roll with jam, and a small bowl of cereal with fruit and low-fat milk; *or,* a half cup plain, vanilla, or lemon yogurt, with a bran or corn muffin and four ounces of orange juice.

Drink only enough coffee or tea to clear your head; then abstain from caffeine, if you can, until late afternoon.

Skip exercise in the morning, even if it is an important part of your daily routine. In fact, try to be as sedentary as possible until just before your flight.

Sleeping late, eating little, and avoiding caffeine and physical activity in the morning will all help trick your biological clock into functioning more as it would if you lived in a westerly time zone, where it is still too early in the morning to be up and around.

For the same reason, delay lunch until after two o'clock, if you can manage it. This meal should be small, too—just a sandwich made with three to four ounces of low-fat protein, and perhaps a piece of fruit. Don't drink coffee or tea at lunch unless you are a caffeine addict and simply cannot do without it.

Do not have a midafternoon carbohydrate snack even if you are accustomed to one. It will initiate serotonin production and put you in a more relaxed state of mind, which, for anti–jet lag purposes, you should avoid until much, much later in the day.

At four or five o'clock, when your biological rhythms have peaked and are beginning to proceed through the stages that will ready you for sleep—but when inhabitants of time zones to the west are gearing up for the busiest part of their day—have a cup of coffee or tea. If you haven't had caffeine for several hours, this cup will pack more power than otherwise, jolting your brain and your body to alertness and ever so slightly retarding the progress of your biological clock.

Now, or just before you leave for the airport, is also a good time to get in some exercise. Vigorous activity late in the day will keep your metabolic rate higher longer into the evening— important because overcoming jet lag quickly requires that you delay nocturnal metabolic slowdown.

On the Plane

The number of meals you will be served in flight obviously depends on how long you will be airborne. Typically, your first meal en route will correspond to the one you would be eating if you were still at home. In other words, if your plane departs in late afternoon, flight attendants will have dinner ready at the normal time for this meal in your home zone. As you move closer to your destination, meals and their timing will be shifted gradually so that they are more in accord with the eating schedule in your new westerly time zone.

The most effective way to deal with what will seem to your mind and body to be inappropriate meals served at peculiar hours is simply to choose foods that will help you stay awake as long as possible. Pick out the protein portions of each meal and eat them first, along with any vegetables, low-fat dairy products, and unsweetened fruit that may be served. High-protein eating will, of course, aid you in your attempts to stave off sleep.

In addition to starting your meals with protein, keep carbohydrate intake low by avoiding foods such as rolls, crackers, bread and breadsticks, carbohydrate appetizers, and sweet or starchy desserts.

Since fatty foods, like carbohydrates, induce postmeal drowsiness, do not eat high-fat meats such as sausage or pâtés; creamy, oily, or cheese-based sauces, toppings, and salad dressings; cheese snacks and dips; stuffed eggs; vegetables drenched in butter or served with mayonnaise; and rich desserts.

Of course, avoid all alcohol until you are ready to sleep.

If coffee or tea tends to keep you awake, take advantage of that fact during your flight. Although it is in general a good idea to keep caffeine intake low, an extra cup or two of your favorite beverage at nine or ten in the evening on an east-to-west flight won't hurt, and it should delay drowsiness, which is the primary aim of this anti–jet lag strategy.

Physical activity will also help keep you awake. It's impossible to do anything really strenuous on a jumbo jet, but you *can* take an occasional walk up and down the aisle. If aisles are constantly blocked by serving carts, then at least change position in your seat from time to time. Even small movements such as these will make a difference!

Once You Have Landed

Upon arrival, adhere as closely as possible to the normal
meal pattern in your destination time zone. For a while, until
your mind and body adjust to the new schedule, you will be
out of sync. You may have little or no appetite for some meals,
especially those that occur at times when you would be
sleeping if you were home. And you will be hungry at inopportune hours—in the middle of the night, for example. You will
feel a tremendous desire to sleep in the afternoon and, perhaps, to spring out of bed at two, three, or four in the morning,
ready to start a new day. Nevertheless, you *will* adapt, and
you will do so more quickly and easily if you make the effort
to conform to local custom and continue to follow anti–jet lag
guidelines.

Which Foods When

As you might expect, the basic rule for anti–jet lag eating
when traveling from east to west (note that Japan and China
are west when flying from the United States) is an inverted
version of the rule for west-east eating: Have a high-carbohydrate breakfast. Follow it with a lunch and dinner that emphasize protein.

Why morning carbohydrates? Because, if you have crossed
many time zones to arrive at your destination, it is quite likely
that you will awaken at an inappropriately early hour. Carbohydrates in the early morning may help you delay to a later
hour the full revving up of your biological rhythms. Remember, to kick jet lag faster in a time zone west of your own, you
must make a conscious effort to sleep longer—or at least be
quiescent in the early morning—and to stay up later at night.

As for high-protein lunches and dinners, they will contribute to your ability to stay awake and active in the afternoon
and evening.

The specific food strategies to use in coaxing your internal clock to wake you up later, and keep you awake later, are as follows:

BREAKFASTS. Waking up much too early is perhaps the most disorienting aspect of travel from east to west. One client told me that on the first day of a recent week-long business trip to Japan, his eyes snapped open at 3 A.M. (Tokyo time), and although he tried, he simply could not go back to sleep. His body, of course, was still running on home zone time. He did what to him seemed wise under the circumstances: He got into his running clothes and took the elevator down to the hotel's outdoor track. "What was almost as weird as finding myself running at three in the morning was seeing five or six other Americans out there jogging in the dark," he said.

Not only will you probably awaken at the time you ordinarily get up at home—in the middle of the night or predawn in your destination time zone—it is also likely that your appetite will be hearty and that you will want a gigantic breakfast.

Hold off for as long as possible. Get back into bed and see if you can manage to fall asleep again. (Better still, don't even get out of bed.) If you find you can't sleep, do something quiet that requires a minimal expenditure of energy—read or watch television. *Do not get up and exercise,* as my client did. Any strenuous activity now will reinforce the tendency of your biological clock to continue operating on home zone time.

When hunger becomes insistent, have a light, high-carbohydrate breakfast of juice; cereal; and bread, toast, a roll, bagel, or muffin with jelly instead of butter to further boost the carbohydrate content of the meal.

Avoid caffeine for now—it will further rev up your brain and body and thus prolong the period of adjustment. If you want something hot with breakfast, order decaffeinated coffee or tea.

Drink the juice, then read or watch more television for a while before you start on the rest of your food. Stretch the meal out for as long as possible so that when you finish, it will be close to the normal breakfast hour in your new time zone.

Juice and toast or a muffin don't make much of a breakfast, especially when, in your old time zone, you'd be thinking about lunch. So you probably will be hungry throughout the morning. If so, nibble on something light, such as fruit and crackers, at midmorning, but don't have a real meal until lunchtime.

Delay your first cup of coffee or tea as long as you can—at least until seven or eight o'clock, the breakfast hour in your new time zone, which also corresponds to the time when mental and physical energy levels begin to slide at home. The caffeine will help sharpen your thought processes and increase alertness—important if you have sales calls to make or meetings to attend. (Even if you plan to spend the day sight-seeing, the mental energy boost provided by caffeine will heighten your awareness and appreciation of unfamiliar surroundings.)

LUNCHES. At midday in your new time zone you will be ready for a big meal, since—depending on how far you have traveled from your home zone—your biological clock will now be sending out signals that it is well past dinner time.

You will adapt much more quickly to local schedules if you keep this meal smallish—"lunch-size." Overeating now will promote drowsiness afterward, and unless you have time for an afternoon nap, your desire to sleep will only increase as the day progresses. Result: You may find yourself forced to turn in at five or six in the evening, and the entire out-of-sync cycle will begin all over again the next morning, when once again you awaken well before the dawn.

You can begin lunch with a neutral food (one that will not trigger the production either of the alertness chemicals *or* the calming chemical). Clear soups, fruit, and nonstarchy vegetables are all neutrals. Or start it with four to five ounces of protein, such as fish, other seafood, poultry, veal, or lean beef. A chef's salad would also be good, but only if it is *lightly* dressed. (If you ask for dressing on the side, you will be able to control the amount.) Tuna, shrimp, or chicken salad platters are safe, too, if they contain little or no mayonnaise.

Avoid fats in general so that you won't feel drowsy as a result of calorie overload. Even relatively modest amounts of heavy gravy, rich, creamy sauces and soups, butter on vegetables and bread, etc., can produce the mental and physical slowdown you must guard against now. (Finding low-fat meals shouldn't be a problem if you are in the Far East, since traditional Japanese, Chinese, and Korean cuisines tend to be low in fat. But be careful when you dine in restaurants featuring Continental or American food.)

Keep carbohydrate intake low. Limit yourself to just a nibble of bread or roll or a couple of bites of rice, potato, or noodles. Even these small amounts of carbohydrate should be eaten *after* you have finished the protein component of your meal.

Drink no alcohol at lunch. You may not fully recover from its sedative effects until two or three o'clock tomorrow morning, unless you can manage to take a nap this afternoon—an excellent idea, as I will explain shortly.

No dessert, unless it is unsweetened fruit. Fruit served in syrup or otherwise sweetened will counter some of the brain-rousing effects of your protein main course.

Finish lunch with a cup or two of coffee or tea. It will help maintain mental alertness, which may be flagging now, since, depending on how far away from home you are, it is evening—perhaps even bedtime—according to your biological clock.

P.M. SLEEP/EXERCISE BONUS. Expect your level of energy to take a nosedive sometime in the afternoon on the first two or three days in a time zone west of where you live. There is a perfectly logical reason for this dip: It's bedtime or later back home.

A short nap will help you recoup partially—mentally and

physically—and should enable you to stay awake until a reasonable hour for bed in your new time zone. Don't nap for more than an hour. Set your alarm clock, or ask the hotel front desk for a wakeup call so you won't continue sleeping through the evening and into the wee hours of the next day. (If that happens, you will in effect have retained your home zone sleep schedule and be back to square one with regard to shaking off jet lag.)

If you can arrange for a brief period of exercise after your nap, so much the better. A brisk fifteen- to twenty-minute walk or slow jog, fifteen minutes on a stationary bike, or a few laps in the hotel pool will bring your body temperature and metabolism back up to daytime levels and thus help set your biological clock to a sleep/wake cycle closer to normal for your new time zone.

Avoid all carbohydrates now. You will probably be ravenous for sweets or starches late in the afternoon. That is your system's way of fooling you into getting your brain to make more sleep-inducing serotonin. (Remember, it is night back home.) If you give in, you may as well cancel any meetings or social engagements planned for the evening. Although you might be physically able to get where you want to go, your mind will be off in dreamland! If you are truly hungry now, have some protein or a protein-carbohydrate combination snack, such as cottage cheese and a couple of crackers. Neither will satisfy your specific craving for carbohydrates, but protein (or protein and carbohydrate together) will do something far more useful: By inhibiting serotonin production, it will help put a speedier end to jet lag.

If, despite nap, exercise, and a protein-based snack, you nevertheless feel your brain beginning to fog, have a cup of coffee or tea.

DINNERS. Remember, *when* you eat is as important as *what* you eat. In combatting east-to-west jet lag, it is imperative that you delay dinner for as long as possible. After all, you can't sleep while you eat. Therefore, if you can postpone the meal until at least seven, you know you will still be awake at eight.

Like lunch, dinner should be a high-protein meal with little or no carbohydrate and should consist of light, easy-to-digest foods. Your system is still on home zone time, which means your internal clock is set for sleep, and a heavy meal now may make you feel distinctly uncomfortable.

Here are the specifics: Ignore rolls, bread, or breadsticks if they are placed on the table before you order. Have a small protein or low-fat vegetable appetizer and follow it with a low-fat entrée such as baked fish or a clam or fish chowder, some other seafood, chicken, a beef or veal stew (well trimmed of fat), or even scrambled eggs. Round out your meal with a salad or a serving of a leafy green or bright-colored vegetable. Take only two or three bites of rice, noodles, pasta, or potato if they come with your order. Once again, unsweetened fruit is the only safe choice for dessert.

Do *not* have alcohol before, during, or after your meal.

Do have coffee or tea at its conclusion. Caffeine, if you can tolerate it at all, will be one of your most useful tools in dealing with the afternoon-into-evening brain drain that characterizes east-to-west jet lag. (Yes, I have been advising more coffee and tea here than in other chapters, and some of you may prefer not to drink as much as I have suggested. Naturally, if you find that you can function at or near peak mentally and physically without increasing your caffeine intake, disregard my advice. But if you feel slowed-down and draggy despite following all the other anti–jet lag guidelines, try getting more caffeine into your system at the times I have indicated. It might make all the difference. You won't need to maintain such high caffeine levels after a couple of days, when jet lag symptoms disappear.)

BEDTIME. Your main problem in the evening will be to stay awake until an appropriate hour for bed in your new time zone. It won't be easy, especially on the first day after you land, when your system will be fighting hardest to maintain home zone sleep patterns.

Nevertheless, *force* yourself to stay awake until at least nine-thirty or ten. If you are successful—and you will be if you try hard enough—the chances of your awakening at two, three, or four in the morning will be greatly reduced. And so will your jet lag symptoms!

My west-to-east and east-to-west anti–jet lag strategies work. Although they won't "cure" jet lag—only time will do that—they *will* significantly speed your adjustment to a new time zone. And, given the changed circumstances, they will keep you as mentally sharp and energetic as it is possible to be and thus add immeasurably to the success and/or pleasure of your trip.

However, as I mentioned before, even if you follow anti–jet lag strategies to the letter, it is still a good idea to plan your trip so that you won't have to rise to the demands of important business or social obligations at times when you are apt to feel most fatigued and out of it. For west-to-east travelers, the first mornings are the critical periods. East-to-west travelers will be hit hardest in the afternoon and evening.

I've known Europeans, for example, who plan on attending dinner parties, Broadway shows, and other evening events just hours after arriving in the United States. Not too long ago, one of them sat next to me at a concert, having insisted beforehand that just because he had flown in from Germany that afternoon didn't mean he wasn't up to enjoying the works of his favorite, Mozart. Fortunately, the music masked his snores.

13. Eating
to Ease Stress

"Eat, you'll feel better."

Who hasn't heard that advice dozens of times from parents, relatives, concerned friends? As advice goes, it's quite good. Food really does have the potential to make you feel better when you are upset, worried, anxious, frustrated, tense. In fact, the more my colleagues and I study the subject, the more convincing is the evidence that the right food, eaten in moderation, is among the most effective and safest of all stress relievers.

Food is certainly better at easing acute, temporary feelings of stress than either cigarettes or alcohol—and has none of their harmful side effects. In fact, the right food at the right time in the right amount is as effective as a tranquilizer—and is better for you, since these drugs, like tobacco and alcohol, are potentially harmful and subject to abuse.

The stress-relieving effect of food can be *so* pronounced and immediately apparent that at least one volunteer participant in the food/mind/mood studies carried out at M.I.T. was convinced that we (the scientists overseeing the project) had put a mind-altering drug in his lunch. When asked why, he replied that it was inconceivable to him that any food could make him feel as relaxed and mellow as he did after he finished his meal!

But it was food and food alone that had caused the remarkable change in his mood. More specifically, it was carbohydrate food.

The biological mechanism that triggers stress—a blanket term used here to cover a range of negative feelings, from anger to worry to anxiety to tension to frustration—is still not completely understood. However, there is evidence that in a stressed state the brain more quickly uses up its supply of the chemicals that dictate emotions and state of mind. When the brain begins to make more serotonin, as it does when carbohydrates are eaten, negative feelings are eased; anger is moderated, worrisome problems seem to shrink in magnitude, the edge is taken off anxiety, tension diminishes, and it becomes easier to deal with frustration.

Eating carbohydrates takes the immediate pressure off long enough to enable you to stand back and consider more rationally and coolly the options for dealing with the *cause* of your stress.

In this chapter, I am going to tell you how to eat to ease acute, episodic stress—the kind you experience when a report is misplaced, an order is canceled, a tire goes flat and makes you late for a meeting or date, a colleague gets credit for work that *you* did, or you fail to meet a deadline. I am not going to deal here with long-term chronic stress, such as that brought about by a lingering illness, ongoing marital problems, months of joblessness, etc. Although food may help lessen the day-to-day emotional pain and discomfort of chronic stress, it won't change the circumstances that cause the stress. Only professional intervention and/or hard work on your part will do that.

The Carbohydrate "Cure" for Acute Temporary Stress

I always ask clients what they eat when they are upset. More often than not they'll say, "Anything," or "Whatever I can get my hands on." But when I probe further and ask for recent examples, the foods named are almost invariably carbohydrates. Nature, it seems, has a way of guiding us to sweets and starches when we are feeling stressed.

But nature doesn't tell us which *kinds* of sweets and starches to eat in order to get the relief we are looking for. Or *how* to eat these foods to obtain the greatest benefits. Or the "dosage" required to do the job. Or when to *stop* eating, in order to avoid calorie overload and unwanted weight gain.

Recent research at M.I.T. and elsewhere has yielded answers that nature didn't supply. And client after client has attested to the success of the stress-easing food strategies developed on the basis of that research.

For sure, safe relief from feelings of acute temporary stress, these are the guidelines to follow:

Eat Carbohydrate Alone, Unaccompanied by Protein

As I have mentioned many times, the amino acids supplied by protein prevent tryptophan from getting to the brain, so that calming serotonin will not be manufactured in amounts large enough to ease stress.

Do not do as one of my clients did after I suggested that he eat some carbohydrate to relax after one of his frequent run-ins with the boss. He got a roast beef sandwich from the office vending machine. Bread, he reasoned, and quite correctly, is a carbohydrate food. But he forgot the other, equally important point—avoid protein. No wonder he was somewhat chagrined by the lack of results . . . and told me so on his next visit.

When you want to combat negative feelings brought on by

stress, it is imperative that your carbohydrate "cure" be unmixed with protein.

Low-fat Carbohydrates Offer Quickest Stress Relief

Fatty accompaniments make many carbohydrates taste better. We put butter on bread, sour cream on a baked potato, cream cheese on a bagel, and cheese on crackers because these combinations are delicious. But it is not taste that relieves tension, anger, anxiety, or frustration, despite the fact that some of my clients—and perhaps you, too—believe that flavor is a factor. (One client, for example, used to comfort herself with cream puffs, claiming they were the only food that made her feel better. However, she finally admitted that after finishing off several of them she didn't really feel calmer and more relaxed. In fact she felt logy, slightly sick to her stomach, and guilty because of all the extra calories she had consumed. In overeating her favorite comfort food, she exchanged feelings of stress for other, equally negative feelings!)

Experiments prove that increased serotonin, and not taste, is the real promoter of stress reduction. And, as you know, carbohydrates lowest in fat work fastest. Carbohydrate foods with high-fat ingredients take as long as forty-five minutes to an hour to achieve results. (For an extensive listing of low-fat carbohydrate foods that are ideal for quick relief of stress, see Appendix A.)

Eat the Proper "Dosage"

Although no cracker box bears instructions saying "take four and wait twenty minutes for relief," the amount of carbohydrate you must eat in order to activate the serotonin-manufacturing process in your brain is almost as specific as the number of aspirins you must take for a headache or the amount of antibiotic prescribed for a strep throat.

And what is that precise amount? A "dose" of about one and one-half ounces (30 grams) of pure carbohydrate is enough to induce your pancreas to release a quick surge of insulin, which in turn will start the complex process by which soothing serotonin is produced. (Two ounces of gumdrops, three ounces of jelly beans, or two cups of Cheerios supply about 30 grams of carbohydrate.)

If you are considerably overweight, however, your carbohydrate-insulin-tryptophan relief system may be inefficient (a condition that is remedied by weight loss) and you may need to eat as much as two or two and a half ounces (45–60 grams) of pure carbohydrate to obtain quick stress relief. In any event, if the smaller dosage doesn't produce results within twenty minutes, try again with a second, similar dose of carbohydrate, and stay with that dosage.

Don't be discouraged if relief isn't instant. Just as it takes a while for aspirin to make a headache fade away, it will take several minutes after eating carbohydrates before you begin to feel more relaxed and composed, and for the same reason: The carbohydrate, whether it be a cookie, a potato, or a small portion of rice, needs to pass through your stomach and into your small intestine before it can be absorbed into the bloodstream and processed to start up serotonin production. This takes about twenty minutes, more or less, depending on how slowly or rapidly your digestive organs process food.

There are still other factors that can affect how slowly or quickly stressed feelings will disappear after you eat carbohydrates: the fat content of the carbohydrate, the fiber content of the carbohydrate (like fat, high-fiber foods also move more slowly through the digestive tract), and the relative fullness of your stomach and intestine (if either contain food from a previous meal, relief will be slower in coming).

And, if your responses to stress are visceral—i.e., if your stomach clamps shut and your digestion slows almost to a standstill when you are feeling intense anxiety, anger, frustration, etc.—it may take a very long time indeed for carbohydrates to move through to where they can be absorbed into the bloodstream. In fact, you may not feel the calming, relaxing effects until an hour or more after your carbohydrate snack.

Speedier Stress Relief for Visceral Types

How do you know if your response to stress is visceral, so that your digestion slows in times of stress? The signs are easy enough to recognize. You will experience a sensation of fullness or heaviness in your abdomen even though it has been a while since you last ate. And the idea of putting more food into your stomach—even in amounts as small as one or two ounces—will be unappealing and may even make you nauseous.

The fastest, most effective method of "getting" carbohydrates into your system if you suspect your reaction to stress is visceral is to *drink* them. Sip a cup of herb tea with two full tablespoons of sugar mixed into it, or a cup of instant cocoa or hot chocolate (made with water, not milk), or very slowly drink eight ounces of a caffeine-free regular (nondietetic) soft drink.

Take Your Time

I have asked many clients to describe their eating behavior under stress, and I have discovered that most of them react in basically the same way: After the upsetting incident, they reach for food—usually carbohydrates. Then they eat and eat and eat until they feel stuffed and the box or bag or carton that contained the food is empty. Total time from beginning to end of food episode: about five minutes.

When I ask how they feel after one of these brief but intense bouts of eating, the answer is almost always "guilty." And if I then ask whether the guilt adds to or subtracts from the stress they have been experiencing, the answer is, "Guilt *adds* to the stress." And finally, when I ask why they ate so much, they tell me that they didn't start to feel better until they had consumed the last of the dozen cookies, the final teaspoon of the quart of ice cream, or the single remaining slice of pie.

We know from laboratory and clinical studies that *it is always the first one or two cookies, bites of ice cream, or piece of pie—not the last—that initiates the production of serotonin.* So, although results may not be felt until the last bite is eaten, it is the first few bites that are responsible for starting the process and ultimately for providing relief.

To avoid overeating and potential weight gain, it is important not to eat too quickly and to stop immediately when you have consumed the proper carbohydrate "dosage." After that, relax or get busy with something unrelated to food. Relief is on its way. Excessive carbohydrate intake won't make you feel better faster, but it may very well make you fatter!

Rx for Quicker Results

The liquid carbohydrate strategy I recommended for visceral types is also especially useful if you are the sort of person who finds it very difficult to wait for results, and who might continue to eat until guilt, an overstuffed stomach, or stress relief—whichever occurs first—finally puts an end to the binge. Since liquids pass more easily through the stomach, the relaxing effects of carbohydrates in liquid form will be felt sooner than those of carbohydrates that must first be chewed and swallowed.

One more helpful hint: If you sip your liquid carbohydrate through a straw, pausing for a moment or two between sips, you will be surprised at how little you actually need to drink in order to feel mellower, more benign, and at peace with yourself and the world.

Set the Scene for Relaxation

Finally, it is important that you reinforce the stress-relieving properties of a carbohydrate snack by eating it in a calm, relaxed manner, if possible, and in serene and peaceful surroundings.

To use the aspirin-and-headache analogy one more time, when your head throbs with pain, you probably take aspirin, then lie down if you can and reduce the noise level in your room by closing the door. If you are at work when a headache strikes, you take aspirin and then perhaps take a short break, maybe go outdoors (or stand near an open window) for a breath of fresh air. Lying down, shutting out noise, inhaling fresh air—none of these actions make the headache go away, but they *will* enhance the pain-relieving properties of the aspirin. They will also make you more aware of a reduction in your pain when it comes.

In the same way, slowly eating or sipping your carbohydrate stress reliever and then taking a few minutes off to relax will maximize the calming effects of serotonin and will, at the same time, heighten your perception of the easing away of anger, frustration, anxiety, and other negative feelings.

To obtain the best tranquilizing results from carbohydrate foods, do the following:

- Select your carbohydrate, then sit down in a calm, comfortable atmosphere to enjoy it. Do *not* run to the grocery store, refrigerator, or office vending machine for food, tear open the wrapping, if any, and wolf down your carbohydrate on the spot. Frantic eating behavior such as this will only prolong tension.
- Eat slowly. As I emphasized earlier in this chapter, eating too quickly usually leads to eating too much, and the resulting guilt you may feel will offset the stress-relieving effects of your carbohydrate snack.
- Try to do something enjoyable while you eat. If you are at

home, turn on the radio or television or go outdoors and sit quietly in the sun for a few minutes. If you are at work, leaf through a magazine (but only one that is *unrelated* to your job—no professional journals, house organs, or other publications that will keep you anchored in the upsetting here and now), or simply spend a few moments staring out the window.

A brief period of quiet after you eat carbohydrates will help boost the mood-altering effects of the serotonin as it is being synthesized in your brain. It will also give you an opportunity to contemplate the cause of your agitation and to decide on a rational basis what to do about it.

I have a client who told me she used to come home on Friday evenings feeling extremely anxious about the work left undone at her office—work that requires intense mental effort. "On those Fridays," she explained, "I would walk in the door, head immediately to the kitchen, and eat myself practically into a stupor.

"Now I know better. I spread strawberry jam on three or four rice cakes, make myself a cup of herb tea, carry it all into the living room on a tray, and settle into my favorite chair to read as I eat. In less than half an hour I feel much more relaxed.

"But the best part is that by the time I calm down, I am already beginning to formulate new and better approaches to the work I left on my desk . . . and I am also able to forgive myself for not being superhuman. My tolerance for frustration increases as my anger at myself diminishes!"

This client isn't unusual. Her experience mirrors that of dozens of others who have followed these strategies for easing acute temporary stress and who found—to their great relief—that they work! Take it from me: Eat, you'll feel better . . . if the food you choose is one of the low-fat carbohydrates listed in Appendix A.

Priming the "Calmness Pump"

In addition to using carbohydrates to calm yourself in a stressful situation, you also can use them to arm yourself *in advance* for an upcoming ordeal! Although doing so won't remove the source of the stress, it will make your feelings about the event more manageable and enable you to act in a more assured, calm, and rational manner. In fact, I call this tactic "priming the calmness pump."

Let's say, for example, that you are scheduled to attend what is sure to be a highly contentious meeting. Half an hour before the meeting begins, eat a bagel with jelly, sip a non-dietetic soft drink, or have any of the low-fat carbs listed in Appendix A. Then sit back and try to make your mind a blank for fifteen minutes. Spend the next few minutes going over your notes or rehearsing what you want to say at the meeting.

By the time you leave your office for the meeting, your anxiety level will be substantially lowered. And though you may not be totally unruffled as you walk through the conference room door, you will be more composed and better able to speak and act in a reasoned, calm manner, even as your colleagues and coworkers bristle at each other all around you!

Or you may have to face firing someone or deal with an unpleasant family conflict. Whatever it is, try this strategy next time you must face the unfaceable.

How to Use Carbs to Ease All-Day Stress

As we have seen, food can help us better endure and deal with temporary bouts of tension, frustration, anger, and other negative feelings. It can be an equally useful tranquilizing agent in helping us get through longer periods of stress.

I have a client, a scientist, who must spend several weeks each year writing proposals to secure federal funding for research carried out at the university with which he is associated. It is a part of his job that he detests. He tells me that he works himself up into such a state before he begins a proposal that he becomes impossible to live with. And on the day he starts to write, he awakens with his nerve ends quivering, feeling as if there were a lead weight in his stomach.

Although this man is normally very food-conscious and concerned about eating a healthy, well-balanced diet, his food intake changes drastically when he writes. Last time he worked on a proposal, he ate waffles and maple syrup for breakfast, then skipped lunch but nibbled on gumdrops and licorice sticks until dinner, which was a large bowl of mashed potatoes. Just before bed, he made himself a cup of hot chocolate and topped it off with marshmallow fluff!

Peculiar? Yes, but his day-long diet of carbohydrates works to diminish the tension and anger he feels while toiling at a job he hates. The carbohydrates also keep him focused on his writing, making him less vulnerable to distractions that might tempt him away from his work.

I am not going to advise you to eat exactly as this scientist does when he has to force himself to do a job he loathes. But I am going to suggest that you nibble on low-fat, high-carbohydrate foods—and little or nothing else—the next time you must somehow get through a particularly stress-filled twelve or fourteen hours.

The reason for day-long carbohydrate nibbling has to do with the fact that the longer you are psychologically stressed, the greater are the demands on your brain to manufacture more calming serotonin. And the more serotonin available to your brain cells, the better able you will be to deal with anger, frustration, worry, and anxiety . . . and to face up to and successfully master the challenge, whatever it may be.

But, as one client said to me, "If I actually did as you advise, I would look like a blimp—a tranquil blimp, but a blimp all the same."

Not so. Take another look at what my scientist client ate on the day he wrote his latest proposal and notice that he didn't have a single real meal. In fact, his total calorie intake was less than what he normally has.

All-day nibbling on low-fat carbs with frequent breaks for exercise, if possible, is the key to working your way through a stressful day without neglecting obligations and responsibilities—and without putting on an ounce of excess weight.

An Eating Plan for All-Day Stress Relief

The following food guidelines will help you stay calmer, cooler, and more collected on difficult days and thus enable you to achieve your best potential in the task you have set for yourself.

In reading through the guidelines, you will see that eating for all-day stress relief requires that you break a few of the time-honored rules of good nutrition. Don't worry about it. Adhering to these suggestions for one or even two days won't lead to nutritional deficiencies, especially if you take a good multivitamin and mineral supplement each morning.

But do keep in mind that *this plan is not meant to be followed indefinitely for days or weeks at a stretch.* If you feel intolerably stressed on most days, I urge you to seek the help of a mental health professional. It is doubtful that your problems or your performance will be helped by food.

• *Skip meals; snack instead!* When I first mention this rule to clients wanting to know how they can coast through stressful days more easily and more productively, many of them are shocked. Some insist that they must have three good meals a day or they will feel famished, which is stressful in itself. Hunger *is* stressful. But every one of my clients, after giving the matter some thought, realized that on particularly difficult days, not only do they eat three square meals, they also nibble constantly between meals.

Sound familiar? It should. Constant nibbling under stress is practically universal human behavior.

However, if you nibble constantly and eat regular meals as well, your calorie intake may double or even triple (depending on what kind of food you consume) over what is normal and healthy for you.

If a choice must be made—and it must, if you care about your weight—dispense with the meals on difficult days, and instead encourage your brain continuously to make ample amounts of serotonin by judicious nibbling.

• *Nibble on lowest-fat or no-fat carbs.* Among the very best of the minimal-fat carbs are "finger foods," which not only supply what you need to calm down, but also provide important hand-to-mouth gratification, which helps to relieve stressful feelings.

Good choices are:

Air-popped popcorn
Rice cakes
Cheerios and other dry breakfast cereals, used as nibbles
Miniature marshmallows

Stock up on them when you anticipate an all-day siege
• *Include some foods that provide oral gratification.*

Like hand-to-mouth movements, sucking, sipping, and chewing tend to calm and relax. Behavioral scientists don't know exactly why this should be so, but there is speculation that these actions and the comfort they provide are carried over from infancy. As adults, we do not suck our thumbs, but we still derive oral pleasure from smoking, sucking beverages through a straw, and chewing. Thus, low-fat foods that can be sucked or sipped or that require a good deal of chewing are important elements of a stress-relieving regimen.

For easing negative feelings related to stress, then, I advise clients to lay in a good supply of sucking foods, such as:

Lollipops
Popsicles
Sour balls

Ice chips are also excellent for this purpose. Although they won't induce your brain to make serotonin, because the carbohydrate content of water is zero, neither do they supply calories—a definite plus.

For sipping through a straw, try:

Ice water
Iced herb tea, with or without sugar
Iced decaffeinated coffee, with or without sugar
Club soda
Fruit juices

For chewing gratification, you can munch on:

Licorice sticks
Slightly stale bagels broken into bite-size pieces
Shredded Wheat nuggets
Dried fruit rolls (made of fruit pounded flat and rolled up in clear plastic)
Crunchy vegetables, such as raw snow peas, carrots, cauliflow-erets, celery, chunks or shreds of raw cabbage, cucumber *with* the skin. (Since vegetables are neutral foods and do not induce your brain to manufacture serotonin, they are best eaten *after* you have begun to feel the calming influence of carbohydrates.)

Morning-to-Midnight Stress-Easing Strategy

Now that you know what kinds of foods help to ease away anger, anxiety, frustration, and tension—and why—here's how to integrate them into a day's worth of stress-relieving eating.

If, like my grant-writing scientist client, you know in advance that a particular day is likely to be extremely difficult, shop for what you need ahead of time. (If you plan to spend that day at the office, you can cart everything with you—appropriately and safely wrapped, of course—and eat at your desk.)

More often, of course, horrendous days are unanticipated; they just get off to a bad start and go downhill from there. On those days that turn unexpectedly sour, you can switch to my stress-easing food plan at the point when things begin to fall apart. It will see you through and help you do a better job of picking up the pieces.

All-Day Nibble Plan

The most important point to remember about the All-Day Nibble Plan, developed to ease you through a stressful day, is that the foods are meant to be eaten or sipped *slowly*—slowly enough so that each of the following "menus" will last for hours.

MORNING TO NOON

3 pieces fresh fruit, such as bananas, oranges, apples, pears, strawberries, melon, or blueberries, cut into small, bite-size pieces and mixed in a large bowl;

or

2–3 cups of low-calorie cereal to be eaten dry as nibbles—for example, puffed rice or wheat, Cheerios, or Bran or Corn Chex—*mixed with* ½ cup raisins or ½ cup chopped dates

or

Blend together in blender or food processor and sip very slowly:
8 ounces strawberry sorbet *with*
1 cup strawberries *and*
1 tablespoon wheat germ
Eat with:
2–3 rice cakes, broken into small bits

NOON TO MIDAFTERNOON
Mix together in large bowl:
½ cup red cabbage, shredded
½ cup broccoli, sliced
1 cup fresh mushrooms, sliced
1 cup cooked pasta twists
½ cup carrots, sliced
1 cup boiled new potatoes

or

Mix together in a bowl:
1 cup boiled shrimp, cut in bite-sized pieces, *or* 3 ounces white-meat tuna, broken into chunks
¼ cup low-fat braided cheese or skim-milk mozzarella, in bite-sized pieces
½ cup black olives, sliced
Eat with:
1 6″ pita bread, toasted and split in half, *or* 1 toasted bagel, quartered

MIDAFTERNOON TO LATE AFTERNOON
2–3 cups unsalted popcorn *or* 1–2 cups unsalted pretzel sticks
Seltzer or salt-free club soda (sip slowly, as much as you wish)

LATE AFTERNOON TO MIDEVENING
1 cup clear soup (sip slowly to prolong "meal")
Nibble on any two *of the following entrées:*
1 order Chinese barbecued chicken wings
1 order shredded chicken or vegetables in paper-thin pancakes (moo shu–style)
1 order Chinese dumplings (steamed)
3–4 ounces of miniature meatballs
1 cup meat-filled ravioli
1 cup stuffed shells
1 cup cheese- or meat-filled tortellini
4–5 stuffed grape leaves
4 ounces cold chicken or turkey in bite-sized chunks
1 cup potato gnocchi
1 cup plain tube pasta
1 cup tiny new potatoes, cubed
1–2 carrots, 1 red or green pepper, 6 plum or cherry tomatoes, 1 cup string beans, 1 cup cucumber, and 1–2 pickles, cut into bite-sized pieces and mixed together in a large bowl
Sip very slowly:
Hot or iced regular or decaffeinated tea or coffee; seltzer or salt-free club soda, as desired

LATE EVENING
1–2 frozen fruit bars, Popsicles, or low-fat ice milk on a stick, *or*
7–8 marshmallows, *or*
1–2 cups plain or caramel-coated popcorn, *or*
Turkish taffy or other chewy candy. (Place in freezer, crack into small pieces; limit consumption to 1½ ounces every 2 hours.)

Although the All-Day Nibble Plan offers an abundance of foods, your calorie count for the day will remain about what it would be if you ate normal meals and snacks. Yes, you *can* improve your mood with food without worrying about your weight!

Again, please keep in mind that feelings such as anger, anxiety, frustration, and tension are your own emotional responses to unpleasant or disturbing situations or events, and that my stress-relieving food strategies will not change or do away with the source of your discomfort. *If stress is chronic, see a professional.* But if it is an understandable reaction to a temporary upset, then following the guidelines in this chapter will help you feel better and deal better with the problem . . . and allow you to get on with your work and your life.

14. Food/Mind/Mood and Your Future

Recently I told a colleague about my work on this book. He remarked that it couldn't have been written ten years ago. Back then, the idea that there is a connection between food, the brain, and behavior would have been dismissed as an old wives' tale, or it would have been explained away by a psychological theory about mother, chocolate cake, and rewards. Now, however, it seems as if the organizers of every major medical and scientific conference want to include the subject for discussion, and writers for the popular press call me almost every day wanting to know more about how food can improve brain power, manage moods, and modify behavior.

The field of nutrition as it relates to performance and behavior is new, so new that it doesn't have a name yet. It came into being after research confirmed a definite relation between consumption of protein and carbohydrate foods and the increased manufacture and activity of certain brain chemicals. What I have done here is share these discoveries with you and explain how you can apply them to maximize your performance. But you should realize that even as I write this book—and even as you read it—new findings are being reported, new and better ways of understanding how food affects performance and mood are being determined, and new ways of implementing this important information are being developed. So, although this book is accurate and current, do not be surprised to read in a newspaper or other periodical that even more exciting food/mind/mood discoveries have been made.

To give you an idea of what the future may bring, I want to mention some areas not covered in this book in which research is being actively conducted—and from which practical recommendations on new ways to use food to manage your mind and your moods should be forthcoming.

A recent study carried out and published by two pediatricians suggests that serotonin is involved in the process by which newborn infants begin to sleep through the night and stay awake during the day. Of course, these experiments simply confirm what mothers have known since the dawn of history: Carbohydrate helps babies sleep through the night. Still, it is good to begin to understand *why*.

At the other end of the life cycle, we are conducting research here at M.I.T. to see whether carbohydrate or protein foods eaten at different times might be influential in sustaining a high level of performance and an evenness of mood among very old adults. And investigations have been in progress now for many years on whether one constituent of food, lecithin, is beneficial in preventing the deterioration in memory associated with Alzheimer's disease. Although the work has been limited by the difficulty of obtaining pure lecithin (health food store lecithin is very impure), results may be available in the near future.

Premenstrual syndrome is another disorder that may yet be managed by diet. It is known that women who suffer from

PMS experience changes in their mood, in their ability to concentrate and work effectively, and in their energy levels. Since food preferences sometimes change drastically in the days before menstruation, my colleagues and I are doing research to determine whether certain foods ease or exacerbate some of the symptoms.

Seasonal affective disorder is another food and mood related disorder. It is characterized by mild depression that develops in the fall and winter and seems to be triggered by the seasonal decrease in daylight. SAD, as it is called, is spontaneously "cured" in the spring when the days become longer. People who suffer from it complain of having great difficulty functioning at their usual high levels; they perform less well at work and make fewer social and family commitments. Many retire into what appears to be semihibernation. The symptoms are accompanied by a marked increase in appetite, especially for sweet carbohydrates. In our studies on SAD, we are attempting to determine whether some of these symptoms can be alleviated by diet. As of now, the prospects are promising.

As you can see, we are on the verge of many discoveries that may have a direct impact on how you or someone close to you feels, performs, and behaves. I believe that if I were writing this book next year or the year after, I would be able to include the results of much of the current research and thus help you to manage your mind and your moods even better.

But until we know more, use what we already *do* know about the food/mind/mood connection to boost your potential at work and in your personal life, and to bear up better under stress.

Put the food/mind/mood principles into practice. Doing so may be the single most important step toward success you will ever take!

APPENDIX A.
Stress-Easing, Mind-Focusing, Sleep-Inducing High-Carb Snacks

Listed below are snacks containing 200 or fewer calories and enough carbohydrate to increase serotonin production in the brain. Assuming that your weight is about normal for your height and bone structure, eating these snacks in the amounts indicated will help you feel calmer, less stressed, and better able to concentrate during the day. They will also help you get to sleep if eaten shortly before bedtime. If you are more than 20 percent over your ideal weight, you will probably need to eat one-third to one-half more than the amounts listed in order to obtain the desired results.

The list, of course, is not comprehensive. However, it does include many of the prepared snack foods that are available nationwide. If your favorite snack is missing from this list, check the label for its calorie and carbohydrate content, or call or write the quality-control department of the manufacturer and ask for this important information.

Type	Amount	Calories	Carbohydrate (grams)
CANDY			
Candy Corn	2 oz.	203	50.8
Caramels	1.5 oz.	169	32.5
Vanilla or chocolate fudge	1.5 oz.	169.5	32
Gumdrops	2 oz.	196	49.5
Jelly beans	2 oz.	208	53
Marshmallows	2 oz.	180	45.6
Mints	2 oz.	206	51
Charleston Chew	1.5 oz.	179	32.6
Chuckles	2 oz.	184	46
Clark Bar	1.4 oz.	188	28.4
Licorice: Crows or Dots	1.5 oz.	165	40.5
Licorice or cherry bars, bits, or stix	2 oz.	188	44.2
Lollipops (Life Savers)	2 pops, 0.9 oz. each	198	48
Milk Duds (Clark)	2.75 oz.	178	35.6
Peppermint Pattie (Nabisco)	3 pieces, 0.5 oz. each	192	37.5
Mallo Cup (Boyer)	3 0.6-oz. pieces	162	33.6
Spearmint Leaves (Curtis)	6 0.7-oz. pieces	192	48
Sugar Babies (Nabisco)	1.5 oz.	198	42
Sugar Mama (Nabisco)	1.6 oz.	202	37.2
Sugar Daddy (Nabisco)	7 pieces	189	42
Turkish Taffy (Bonomo)	1.5 oz.	162	37
3 Musketeers	2 0.8-oz. bars	198	35
CEREALS			
Alpha Bits	1½ cups	169.5	36.6
Apple Jacks (Kellogg)	1¾ cups	192	45.5
Cracklin Oat Bran (Kellogg)	¾ cup	180	30
Cocoa Puffs (General Mills)	1½ cups	165	37.5
Honey and Nut Sugar Frosted Flakes (Kellogg)	1¼ cups	165	39
Golden Grahams (General Mills)	1½ cups	165	36
Grape-Nuts (Post)	½ cup	215	46
Honey Smacks (Kellogg)	1⅓ cups	168	37.5
Nutri Grain (Kellogg)	¾ cups	156	36
Puffed Rice (Malt-O-Meal or Quaker)	4 cups	200	48
Spoon Size Shredded Wheat (Nabisco)	1⅓ cups	165	35
Sugar Corn Pops (Kellogg)	1½ cups	165	39
Mix 'n Eat Cream of Wheat, regular or flavored	1.25-oz. packet	170	32
Cooked grits	1⅓ cups	168	36
Instant oatmeal (H-O)	1.5-oz. packet	160	31.8
Instant oatmeal (Quaker)			
Maple and Brown Sugar	1.5-oz. packet	163	32
Raisins and Spice	1.5-oz. packet	159	31.4
Cinnamon and Spice	1⅝-oz. packet	176	34.8
COOKIES			
Animal Crackers (Keebler)			
iced	8	192	31.2
regular	16	192	32
Apple Spice (Pepperidge Farm)	4	212	30.4
Apricot Raspberry (Pepperidge Farm)	4	200	30.4
Chocolate Lace and Pirouette (Pepperidge Farm)	5	185	35

Type	Amount	Calories	Carbohydrate (grams)
Bordeaux (Pepperidge Farm)	6	198	32
Brown edge wafer (Nabisco)	7	196	29.4
Butterscotch Chip (Nabisco)	8	192	30
Famous wafer (Nabisco)	7	196	32.2
Snap (Nabisco)	12	192	35
Cinnamon Treats (Nabisco)	7	196	35
Devil's food cake (Nabisco)	2	140	31
Fig Newton (Nabisco)	3	180	33
Fig Wheats (Nabisco)	3	180	34.5
Gingerman (Pepperidge Farm)	6	198	30
Gingersnaps (Nabisco)	6	180	33
Ladyfingers	5	200	35
'Nilla Wafer (Nabisco)	10	190	30
Cookie Little (Nabisco)	33	198	33
Vanilla Cookie Break (Nabisco)	4	200	29.2
Social Tea biscuit (Nabisco)	9	198	31.5
Spiced wafer (Nabisco)	6	198	36

CRACKERS

Type	Amount	Calories	Carbohydrate (grams)
Graham crackers (Nabisco)	12	180	31.2
Graham crackers (Dixie Belle)	12	180	31.2
English Water Biscuit (Pepperidge Farm)	10	170	31.2
Arrow Root Biscuit	10	200	35
Meal Mates (Nabisco)	10	198	29
Milk Lunch Biscuits (Keebler)	7	189	31.5
Oyster Crackers	2 oz.	198	32
Oysterettes or Dandy (Nabisco)	2 oz.	198	32
Royal Lunch (Nabisco)	4	220	32
Rye toast (Keebler)	13	208	27.3
Rye Krisp	8 triple crackers	200	40
Saltines	15	180	30
Sea Rounds (Nabisco)	4	180	30
Sea Toast (Keebler)	3	180	30
Snacks Sticks (Pepperidge Farm)	12	192	30
Soda Gitana (Nabisco)		180	30
Table Water Cracker (Carr's)	6 large	192	35.4
Triscuit (Nabisco)	10	200	30
Uneeda Biscuit (Nabisco)	9	198	33.3
Waldorf (Keebler)	14	196	32
Wheatmeal Biscuit (Carr's)	5 small	210	29.5

STARCHY SNACKS

Type	Amount	Calories	Carbohydrate (grams)
Bagel, plain	1.9 oz.	163	28.3
egg	3″ diameter	162	30.5
Biscuit, Buttermilk—oven ready (Ballard)	4	200	40
Biscuit, regular	4	200	40
Cinnamon Raisin Bread (Thomas's)	3 0.8-oz. slices	180	35.1
Orange and Raisin Bread (Pepperidge Farm)	3 0.9-oz. slices	210	37.5

Type	Amount	Calories	Carbohydrate (grams)
Brown Bread (canned) (B & M)	2 1/2" slices	160	36.4
Blueberry Rounds (Morton)	2 1.5-oz. rounds	220	42
Bran'nola (Arnold)	2.3-oz. muffin	160	30
Cinnamon Raisin English Muffin (Pepperidge Farm)	2-oz. muffin	150	28
Cinnamon Raisin English Muffin (Roman Meal)	2.3-oz. muffin	150	29.8
Raisin English Muffin (Thomas's)	2.2-oz. muffin	153	30.4
Raisin English Muffin (Arnold)	2.2-oz. muffin	170	35
Corn muffin (Morton)	1.9-oz. muffin	180	27
Crumb Bun, French (Sara Lee)	3/4-oz. piece	188	30
Sourdough French roll (Pepperidge Farm)	2 1.3-oz. rolls	200	38
Old Fashioned rolls (Pepperidge Farm)	3 0.6-oz. pieces	180	35
Pan (Wonder)	2 1 1/4-oz. pieces	198	35
Dinner Party Rounds (Arnold)	3 0.7-oz. pieces	165	30
Francisco French bread (Arnold)	2-oz. roll	160	31
Pop-Tart (Kellogg) strawberry	1	200	37
frosted, blueberry or strawberry	1	200	38
cherry chocolate fudge	1	200	36
Toastees (Howard Johnson) blueberry	1	121	48
corn	1	112	51.3
oatmeal	2	190	106.4
orange	1	127	54.8
raisin bran	1	194	55.4
Popcorn dry-popped (Super Pop)	2 oz.	200	40
caramel-coated (Bachman)	1.5 oz.	165	37.5
Pretzels	1 3/4 oz.	192	36.6
Unsalted pretzels (Featherweight)	2.5 oz.	175	32.5
(Rokeach)	1.5 oz.	165	30
MISCELLANEOUS			
Yellow cupcake (Sara Lee)	1	190	31.5
Mr Misty (Dairy Queen/Brazier)	8.25 oz.	190	48
Chocolate sundae (Dairy Queen/Brazier)	3.75 oz.	190	33
Fudgsicle (Popsicle Industries)	2 2 1/3-oz. bars	200	46
Jell-O Pudding Pops	2 2-oz. pops	188	31.2
Rice pudding	1/2 cup	176	30
Danny-in-a-Cup frozen yogurt (Dannon)	8 oz.	180	33

APPENDIX B.
Sample Recipes for Recommended Dishes

CHILI

    2 onions
    2 teaspoons cooking oil
    1½ pounds ground chuck
    1 10½-ounce can tomato soup
    1 1-pound can crushed or whole tomatoes
    1 1-pound can kidney beans
    1 teaspoon chili powder (more if you want it hotter)
    Salt, pepper, and/or red pepper to taste

Chop onions and brown in cooking oil. Add and brown ground chuck. Add rest of ingredients and simmer for one hour.

Serves 4.

ITALIAN DRESSING

 8 tablespoons red wine vinegar
 4 tablespoons cold water
 1 1/2 teaspoons coarse salt
 1 teaspoon sugar
 1 teaspoon freshly ground black pepper
 1/2 teaspoon paprika
 1/8 teaspoon dry mustard

Combine all ingredients in a small deep bowl and beat with a wire whisk until salt and sugar are completely dissolved. Pour into a screwtop jar and close tightly. Shake well before using. Use 1–2 tablespoons per serving—dressing contains only a few calories per serving.

VITELLO TONNATO

 12 ounces of lean veal loin, cut into 8 thin scallops
 4 tablespoons butter
 4 ounces of mushrooms (optional)
 1 tablespoon flour
 1/3 cup canned condensed chicken broth, diluted with
 1/3 cup of white wine or water
 2 medium onions, finely chopped
 3 ounces water-packed white tuna, drained and flaked
 2 tablespoons mayonnaise
 1 tablespoon wine vinegar
 2 tablespoons capers
 Salt and pepper to taste

Put the veal cutlets between two layers of wax paper and pound until very thin. Melt 2 tablespoons butter in large nonstick skillet. Brown mushrooms and remove to platter. Add cutlets and brown on both sides over moderate heat. Do not overcook. Remove veal to platter.

Melt 1 tablespoon butter in small saucepan and blend in flour. Add diluted broth, slowly stirring, and cook until it is smooth and starts to thicken. Remove from the heat and reserve.

Melt remaining butter in small skillet. Add onions and sauté, stirring, until soft. Add the tuna, mayonnaise, vinegar, and half the capers, chopped. Simmer 5 minutes over very low heat. Season to taste with salt and pepper and add mixture to the broth. Simmer the sauce an additional 5 minutes.

Place sauce mixture in a blender or food processor and purée. Spoon the sauce over the veal and mushrooms, and sprinkle with the remaining capers.

Serves 4.

PASTA WITH SEAFOOD AND MUSHROOM SAUCE

1 tablespoon olive oil
4 scallions, chopped
½ pound mushrooms, sliced
2 tablespoons flour
1 cup milk
½ cup clam juice or white wine
4 tablespoons dry sherry
1 teaspoon dry mustard
1 teaspoon curry powder
Salt, pepper, and cayenne to taste
2 egg yolks, slightly beaten
2 tablespoons freshly squeezed lemon juice
6 ounces crab meat
4 ounces cooked shrimp, cut in half
18 medium-sized fresh oysters
4 cups cooked noodles, kept warm

Sauté scallions and mushrooms in oil in large skillet. Sprinkle flour over mixture in skillet and cook, stirring constantly, about 2 minutes.

Combine milk, clam juice or white wine, sherry, mustard, curry, salt, pepper, and cayenne in a small bowl and mix. Add liquid gradually to skillet, stirring constantly, and cook 2 minutes. Stir a little of the hot sauce into the egg yolks, then stir the yolks into the sauce. Blend the lemon juice, crab, shrimp, and oysters into the sauce. Cook until the oysters curl.

Serve over cooked noodles.

Serves 4.

CHINESE POT ROAST

5–6 tablespoons soy sauce
2 tablespoons brown sugar
6 slices fresh ginger root
2 tablespoons plum sauce (optional)
½ cup cold water
3 tablespoons dry sherry
10 ounces lean boneless beef shin or chuck

Combine soy sauce, sugar, ginger, plum sauce, water, and sherry in a mixing bowl. Stir until sugar is dissolved.

Put beef in heavy Dutch oven or heavy pot with tight cover. Pour sauce over beef and bring it to a boil. Reduce heat, cover tightly, and simmer very gently for approximately 2 hours. Turn meat after the first hour; recover tightly and continue cooking.

To serve, slice meat very thin and arrange over cooked Chinese noodles and pour sauce over all.

Serves 2.

STUFFED CABBAGE ROLLS

1 medium savory cabbage
8 ounces ground round steak or 4 ounces ground steak and 4 ounces ground veal
1 medium onion, chopped
½ cup rice (brown, if possible)
3 ounces plus 1 tablespoon canned tomato paste
1 teaspoon ground nutmeg
1½ teaspoons salt
½ teaspoon freshly ground black pepper
1 tablespoon freshly squeezed lemon juice
2 tablespoons brown sugar
¼ cup raisins

Remove leaves from the cabbage and parboil them in water until tender. Drain, and cut off hard stems and core from each leaf.

Combine the meat, onion, rice, 3 ounces tomato paste, nutmeg, salt, and pepper. Blend thoroughly. Divide the meat mix among 8 good-sized leaves. Place mixture on leaf, tuck in the sides, and roll.

Line a 3-quart saucepan with remaining cabbage, place the rolls on top of it, seam sides down, in one layer. Add just enough water to cover. Combine the remaining tomato paste, the lemon juice, sugar, and raisins in a small bowl; mix and stir into the water in the saucepan. Cover tightly and simmer gently 45 minutes. Add water during cooking if necessary.

Serves 2.

ROAST LONDON BROIL

Marinade
2 tablespoons chili sauce
1½ tablespoons Worcestershire sauce
1½ tablespoons vinegar
3 tablespoons sesame oil
1 teaspoon each of thyme, marjoram, basil, rosemary
3 garlic cloves, crushed
1 small onion, minced
1 10½-ounce can beef bouillon
1 tablespoon fresh orange peel, chopped (optional)
1 teaspoon crushed red (hot) pepper (optional)

2½ pounds London broil (uncooked)

Combine all ingredients for marinade, and marinate beef overnight. (Mix well in marinade.) Remove beef from marinade. Place in heavy pan, and roast at 325 degrees until tender, basting frequently with the marinade.

Serves 4. (Plan on serving 4–5 ounces per person.)

WHITE BEAN SOUP

12 small onions, peeled and halved
7 cubes or packets beef bouillon, dissolved in 5½ cups boiling
    water
2 tablespoons olive oil
¼ teaspoon rosemary
3 carrots, peeled and grated
1 20-ounce can white kidney beans, puréed with their liquid
½ teaspoon white pepper
2 tablespoons dry sherry
2 tablespoons chopped chives
4 ounces chopped cooked chicken
Salt to taste

Combine onions and bouillon in a 4-quart stockpot and cook until
onions are tender. Heat oil in skillet, add rosemary and carrots and
cover pan. Heat until soft and then add to onions. Return stockpot to
heat. Add beans, pepper, and sherry to pot and stir. Add the cooked
chicken and chives, and serve.

Serves 4.

BEEF STEW

2 pounds chuck, cut in 1½" cubes
1 large onion, chopped
3 carrots, chopped
2 red peppers, chopped
1 pound mushrooms
2 parsnips, chopped
2 cups of red wine
Salt and black pepper to taste
6 new potatoes, cut in half

Put all ingredients except potatoes in Dutch oven with tight-fitting lid.
Bake at 325 degrees for 1½ hours. Add potatoes and bake another ½
hour.

Serves 6.

LINGUINE WITH SHRIMP SAUCE

3–4 cloves garlic, minced
½ cup olive oil
2 12-ounce cans stewed tomatoes
2 tablespoons chopped parsley
2 tablespoons oregano
Salt and pepper to taste
1 can pitted black olives
2 tablespoons red wine (optional)
1 pound raw shrimp

Sauté the garlic in olive oil until brown. Add the stewed tomatoes, parsley, oregano, salt and pepper, olives, and wine and simmer sauce until thick. Cook shrimp 3–4 minutes and add to sauce.

Serve over cooked linguine, ¾–1 cup per person.

Serves 4.

POTATO SALAD

2 pounds red potatoes, unpeeled
4 eggs, hard-boiled
1 tablespoon wine vinegar
2 tablespoons mustard (Dijon or English)
4 tablespoons chopped dill or chives
Salt to taste
1 teaspoon white pepper
2 teaspoons oregano
¾ cup olive oil
2 6-ounce cans of water-packed tuna
4 scallions, chopped
12 Spanish or black olives, chopped
1 red pepper, chopped

Cook potatoes and eggs and reserve. Put wine, vinegar, mustard, dill or chives, salt, pepper, and oregano in bowl and mix with a whisk. Whisk in olive oil. Cut potatoes when cool and stir them into dressing. Add eggs, tuna, scallions, olives, and red pepper. Refrigerate an hour before serving.

Serves 4.

CHICKEN MOROCCO

½ cup flour
4 tablespoons each curry powder, cumin, and turmeric
1 tablespoon cayenne
1 pound boned chicken, cut in small pieces
1 tablespoon olive oil
1 tablespoon butter
4 onions, chopped
4 garlic cloves, minced
4 slices ginger, sliced thin
½ pound mushrooms, chopped
4 tomatoes, diced
½ cup golden raisins
½ cup dried apricots
½ cup chutney
Salt and pepper to taste

Mix flour, curry, cumin, turmeric, and cayenne. Dredge chicken pieces in mixture and sauté them in melted butter and oil. Set aside.

Add more oil to pan if needed, then add onions, garlic, ginger, mushrooms; cover pan and cook for a few minutes. Add tomatoes, raisins, apricots, and chutney and simmer covered 5–10 minutes. Add chicken, salt and pepper to taste, and simmer for 10 minutes. Serve over rice, ½ cup per person.

Serves 4.

CREOLE FISH CHOWDER

4 cloves garlic, minced
1 chopped onion
1 teaspoon chili pods (optional)
1 cup chopped green or red pepper
1–2 tablespoons olive oil
¼ cup white wine
1 16-ounce can tomatoes
1 pint clam juice

½ cup of parsley, chopped
Salt and black pepper to taste
1 pound flounder, cut into bite-sized chunks
1 pound crab meat

Sauté garlic, onions, chili pods, and peppers in olive oil for 5–8 minutes. Add white wine and cook over medium heat 4 minutes more. Add tomatoes, clam juice, parsley, salt, pepper, and flounder and simmer for 15 minutes on low heat. Add crab meat and simmer 10 more minutes. Serve over rice.

Serves 4.

BAKED FISH *or* SCALLOPS WITH GINGER

1 tablespoon soy sauce or teriyaki sauce
1–2 teaspoons fresh chopped garlic
2 slices fresh ginger, chopped
2 stalks scallions, chopped
4 ounces of haddock or scallops or bluefish or any other fresh fish

Pour soy sauce, garlic, ginger and chopped scallions over fish or scallops. Cover and bake in 350-degree oven for 15–20 minutes or until done.

Serves 1.

Bibliography

This is a short list of some books and articles that describe the scientific background to the material presented in this book. All the references listed here are available in medical libraries.

Christie, J. J., and McBrearty, E. M. T. "Psychophysiological Investigations of Post-Lunch State in Male and Female Subjects." *Ergonomics* (1979), 22:307–323.

Craig, A.; Baer, K.; and Diekmann, A. "The Effects of Lunch on Sensory-Perceptual Functioning in Man." *International Archives Occupation, Environment, Health* (1981), 49:105–114.

Crisp, A. H., and Stonehill, E. *Sleep, Nutrition and Mood.* New York: Wiley (1976).

Fernstrom, J. D., and Wurtman, R. J. "Brain Serotonin Content: Physiological Regulation by Plasma Neutral Amino Acids." *Science* (1972), 178:414–416.

Gibson, C. J., and Wurtman, R. J. "Physiological Control of Brain Norepinephrine Synthesis by Brain Tyrosine Concentration." *Life Science* (1977), 22:1399–1406.

Hartmann, E.; Spinweber, C. L.; and Ware, C. "L-tryptophan, L-leucine, and Placebo: Effects on Subject Alertness." *Sleep Research* (1976), 5:57.

Leathwood, P., and Pollet, P. "Diet-Induced Mood Changes in Normal Populations. *Journal of Psychiatric Research* (1983), 17:147–157.

Lieberman, H.; Corkin, S.; Spring, B.; Growdon, J. H.; and Wurtman, R. J., "Mood, Performance and Sensitivity: Changes Induced by Food Constituents. *Journal of Psychiatric Research* (1984), 17:135–145.

Lieberman, H.; Spring, B.; and Garfield, G. "The Behavioral Effects of Food Constituents: Strategies Used in Studies of Amino Acids, Protein, Carbohydrate and Caffeine." *Nutrition Reviews* (supplement, May 1986), 61–69.

Lieberman, H.; Wurtman, J.; and Chew B., "Changes in Mood After Carbohydrate Consumption Among Obese Individuals." *American Journal of Clinical Nutrition* (1987), volume 44.

Spring, B. "Recent Research on the Behavioral Effects of Tryptophan and Carbohydrate." *Nutritional Health* (1984), 3:55–68.

Spring, B.; Maller, O.; Wurtman, J.; Digman, L.; and Cozolino, L. "Effects of Protein and Carbohydrate Meals on Mood and Performance: Interactions with Sex and Age." *Journal Psychiatric Research* (1983), 17:155–167.

Wurtman, J. "The Involvement of Brain Serotonin in Excessive Carbohydrate Snacking by Obese Carbohydrate Cravers." *Journal of the American Diet Association* (1984), 84:1004–1007.

Wurtman, R., and Wurtman J. "Nutritional Control of Central Neurotransmitters." In: *The Psychology of Anorexia Nervosa*, ed. by K. M. Pirke and D. Ploog, pp. 4–11, Berlin: Springer Verlag (1984).

Wurtman, R., and Wurtman J. *Nutrition and the Brain*, vol. 7. New York: Raven Press (1986).

Index

A

Adrenaline, 18
Albumin, 22
Alcohol, 37
  at business meals, 118–19
  and conference planning, 177–78
  at conferences, 147, 166
  and jet lag, 211, 214, 216, 220, 224, 226
  at lunch, 71–72
  with predinner conference snacks, 163–64
  at preperformance meals, 122
  on test days, 37
Alertness effect, 20
Allergies, and food/mind/mood strategies, 9–10
All-protein diet, and supply of tryptophan, 21
Alzheimer's disease, diet management of, 248
American Medical Association, on food allergies, 9
Amino acids, 19–20, 21, 22
  natural versus bottled, 23–24
Anti–jet lag tactics, 6, 207–27
  east-to-west eating schedule, 217–27
    after landing, 221
    bedtime, 226–27
    breakfasts, 218, 222–23
    caffeine consumption, 218, 219, 223, 225, 226
    dinners, 225–26

    before leaving, 218–19
    lunches, 219, 223–25
    midafternoon snacks, 219
    on the plane, 219–20
  and exercise, 213–14, 218, 220, 225
  west-to-east eating schedule, 208–17
    after landing, 211
    bedtime, 216–17
    breakfasts, 209, 211, 212–14
    caffeine consumption, 209, 210, 213
    dinners, 209, 210, 211, 212, 214–16
    before leaving, 209–10
    lunches, 209, 214
    midafternoon snacks, 209
    on the plane, 210–11
Appetizers
  avoidance list, 114–15
  at banquets, 139–40
  at business meals, 114–15
  at conference dinners, 168
  as predinner snack, 162–65
  recommended list, 115–17
Artichoke hearts, and ease of eating, 118

B

Baked fish/scallops with ginger, 263
Banquets, eating tactics for, 139–41
Beans, as protein source, 25, 115
Bearnaise sauce, 77

Bedtime snacks
  anti–jet lag, 216–17, 226–27
  carbohydrate, 50, 142, 148
  protein, 49, 141–42
  sleep-inducing, 90–92, 142, 170
Beef, as protein source, 25, 26
Beef stew, 260
Beets, in diet, 28
Behavioral tests, for rating perform-
    ance, 16
Beurre sauce, 77
Biological clock, 31, 56–58. *See also*
    Circadian rhythms
  overcoming; *See* Anti–jet lag tac-
    tics; Night workers
Blood sugar
  and food/mind/mood strategies, 10–
    11
  role of insulin in regulating, 22
Bouillon
  for appetizer, 115
  for lunch, 159
Breakfast
  anti–jet lag
    east-to-west, 218, 222–23
    west-to-east, 209, 211, 212–14
  bring-your-own (conference), 148–
    50
  buffet, 152–53
  day-after
    for motivated night worker, 206
    for obligated night worker, 198
  foods to avoid, 64–65
  hurry-up tips, 67
  modified continental, 150–51
  preperformance, 123–29
  reasons for eating good, 59–61
  recommended amounts, 109
  for stay-at-homes, 65–67
  suggested menus, 62–63
  suggestions for good, 61–62
  timing, 61
  what and how much to eat, 61–62
  with get-up-and-go, 58–67
Breakfast test
  for carbohydrate, 40
  for protein, 39
Broccoli, in diet, 28
Business meals, 107–8
  appetizers, 114–15
  breakfasts, 112, 113
    avoiding alcohol at, 118–19
    and caffeine consumption, 112–13,
      120
    choice of foods at, 108–9
    desserts, 119–20
    dinner, 113
    don't arrive hungry, 111–13
    eat protein before carbohydrate,
      113–17
    eat sparingly, 108–11
    lunch, 113
    order "easy" food, 117–18

C

Cafeteria lunches, 158–61
Caffeine, 95–106
  and A.M. coffee factor, 125
  as afternoon pickup, 99–100
  for all-night
    motivated worker, 201–2, 204
    obligated worker, 193, 194, 196
  assessing risks in consuming, 103–6
  and boosting morning performance
    levels, 98–99
  at coffee break, 99, 128–29
  in combination with carbohydrates,
    100
  at conference, 148, 153, 178–80
  controversy over, 95
  at end of dinner, 120
  evening consumption of, 100–1
  and fibrocystic breast disease,
    104–6
  and jet lag
    east-to-west, 218, 219, 223, 225,
      226
    west-to-east, 209, 210, 213
  and mental alertness, 96–106, 125,
    178–80
  and performance level, 135
  and pregnancy, 104
  at preperformance meals, 123, 125,
    126, 127, 140
  sources of, 103
  tolerance for, 101–3
Caffeine addicts, and coffee consump-
    tion, 129
Calming effect, 21–23
Calorie consumption
  and conference meal planning, 174
  and mental alertness, 71, 110

Calorie content, and power eating, 62, 110
Calorie overload, 60–61, 109, 111, 119, 123, 135
Cancer, link of fat to, 29
Carbohydrate(s), 21–23
  amount needed, 29–30
  for bedtime snacks, 90–92
  and the calming effect, 21–23
  at conference breaks, 176–77
  consumption of, as cure for temporary stress, 231–38
  to ease all-day stress, 238–45
  and east-to-west jet lag, 225
  eating in combination with protein, 22
  eating proteins before, 113–17
  effect of, on performance level, 135, 136
  foods with, 26–28
  as predinner relaxer, 162–65
  and sleep induction, 141–43, 148
  testing your food/mind/mood response to, 40, 42, 44, 46, 48, 50
Carbohydrate craver, 51–52
  afternoon coffee break, 162
  afternoon performance, 136
  identification of, 81
  midafternoon snacks for, 83–84
  midmorning snacks for, 127–28
  need for restorative snacks, 81–83, 128
Carbohydrate eaters
  mistakes made by, in distraction messages, 35–36
  reaction times of, 35
Carrots, in diet, 28
Catecholamines, 18
Catered
  breakfasts, 151–52
  lunches, 157–58
    effect of, on performance level, 132–33
Cheerios, as calming food, 15
Cheese, as protein source, 26
Chef's salad, for lunch, 79, 223–24
Chicken, as protein source, 25
Chicken, boneless breasts of, and ease of eating, 117
Chicken Morocco, 262
Chili, 255

Chinese pot roast, 257
Chinese restaurants
  business meals at, 76–77
  conference dinners at, 167
Chinese specialties, and ease of eating, 118
Chocolate, 10, 142
Chopsticks, avoidance of, at business meal, 118
Circadian rhythms. *See also* Biological clock
  definition of, 55
  overriding, 57–58, 59; *See also* Anti–jet lag tactics; Night workers
  power of, 57
  and protein consumption, 59
Cocoa. *See also* Caffeine
  as source of caffeine, 103
Coffee. *See also* Caffeine
  and the coffee break, 99, 127, 128–29
  as source of caffeine, 103
Coffee break
  A.M. conference, 152–53
  afternoon conference, 161–62
  for the all-night worker, 202–3
  caffeine consumption at, 128–29
  drinking coffee at, 99, 127, 128–29
  food at A.M., 61, 67–69
  and the late-morning performance, 127–29
  serving snacks at, 176–77
Coffeeshop. *See also* Restaurants
  breakfast at, 65
Cola-type soft drinks. *See also* Caffeine
  as source of caffeine, 103, 203
Complex carbohydrates, 26, 28
Conference blahs, 145
  causes and cures of, 146–48
Conference breakfasts
  bring-your-own, 148–50
  buffets, 152
  catered, 151–52
  modified continental, 150–51
  at restaurants, 151–52
Conference coffee breaks
  afternoon, 161–62
  A.M., 152–53
  caffeine at, 153

Conference dinners
  on-duty, 167–70
  off-duty, 166–67
Conference lunches
  at cafeteria/restaurant, 158–61
  catered, 157–58
  do-it-yourself, 154–56
  for afternoon effectiveness, 153–61
Conference meal planning, 171–72
  and alcohol, 177–78
  breakfasts, 182
  caffeinated/noncaffeinated beverages, 178–80
  calories, 174
  coffee breaks, 176–77, 182, 184
  dinners, 184–85
  fats, 175
  lunches, 183
  portion sizes, 173–74
  protein, 175–76
  rules for, 173–81
  taking control, 180–81
Consommé
  as appetizer, 115
  for lunch, 159
Corn sweetener, 27
Cottage cheese, as protein source, 25
Cranberry sauce, 190–91
Creative overload, 200
Creole fish chowder, 262–63
Croissants, 151

D

Danish pastry, 127, 151
Decaffeinated coffee/tea, 101
Decaffeinated espresso, 101
Desserts
  for the all-night worker, 201
  at business meals, 119–20
  at preperformance meals, 133
Digestion, 122–23
Dinner meetings, eating tactics for, 138–39
Dinners
  anti–jet lag
    east-to-west, 225–26
    west-to-east, 209–10, 211, 212, 214–16
  and late-night work
    for the motivated worker, 200–1

for the obligated worker, 192–95, 196–97
  menus, 86–88
  recommended amounts, 109
  suggestions for, 84–86
  that keep you going, 84–88
  for unwinding, 88–89
Dinner test
  for carbohydrate, 44
  for protein, 43
Distraction message test, 35
Do-it-yourself
  breakfast, 148–50
  lunch, 154–56
Dopamine
  as alertness chemical, 18–19, 20, 58, 86, 141, 204
  as mood-modifying chemical, 13
  production of, 22, 30, 31
  role of caffeine on manufacture of, 98
  strategy for increasing, 31, 71, 116

E

"Eating around the entrée" tactics, 133
Egg whites, 24
Entraining, 59, 60, 61, 65–66
Ethnic restaurants
  business meals at, 76–78
  conference dinners at, 167
Evening performance, 136–37
  dinner meeting dinner, 138–41
  at home preperformance dinner, 137–38
Exercise
  for the all-night worker, 194–95, 203–4
  and jet lag, 213–14, 218, 220, 225

F

Fake hunger, 127
Farmer's breakfasts, 64
Fasting, effect of, on mental abilities, 133
Fat(s), 25, 26, 28–29
  in bedtime snacks, 91
  in breakfast foods, 64–65
  and conference meal planning, 175
  in lunch foods, 71

Fettucini Alfredo, 132
Fibrocystic breast disease,
  and caffeine consumption, 104–6
Fish, as protein source, 25
Food allergies, effect of food/mind/
  mood strategies on, 9–10
Food and Drug Administration,
  on food allergies, 9
  regulation of amino
    acids as drugs by, 23
Food intake, measuring, 92–93
Food/mind/mood connection, 3–11
Food/mind/mood response
  to control circadian rhythms, 55–93
  dependability of, 30–31
  effect of fat, 29
  interpreting scores, 51–53
  testing, 15–16, 33–50
    bedtime snacks, 49–50
    breakfast, 39–40
    dinner, 43–44
    lunch, 41–42
    midafternoon snacks, 47–48
    midmorning snacks, 45–46
    procedures, 36–38
Food/mind/mood strategies
  and allergies, 9–10
  and blood sugar, 10–11
  effect of, on habits, 7–8
  as fast-acting, 14–15
  and the future, 247–49
  and nutrition, 8–9
  as proven, 15–16
  safety of, 13–16
Food scale, 92–93
French restaurants
  business meals at, 77–78
  conference dinners at, 167
Fructose, 26, 27
  and serotonin production, 180
Fruit
  and the food/mind/mood response,
    27
  for lunch, 159–60

G
Glucose, 26–27
Grapes, consumption of, for the all-
  night worker, 198
Guacamole, 75

H
Habits, effect of food/mind/mood
  strategies on, 8
Hamburger, for lunch, 75, 79
Health food restaurants,
  eating lunch at, 78, 80
Heart disease, link of fat to, 29
High-fiber vegetables, 132
Hollandaise sauce, 77, 132
Honey, 27
Hors d'oeuvres. *See* Appetizers
Hunger, effect of, on performance
  level, 123
Hypoglycemia, and food/mind/mood
  strategies, 11

I
Indoleamine, 18
Inner clock. *See* Biological clock; Circadian rhythms
Insomnia, and caffeine consumption,
  101
Insulin, 26, 28
  need for, in production of serotonin,
    26, 28, 116, 176–77
  role of, in regulating blood sugar, 22
Italian dressing, 256
Italian restaurants
  business meals at, 77
  conference dinners at, 167

J
Japanese restaurants
  business meals at, 77
  conference dinners at, 167
Japanese specialties, and ease of eating, 118

K
Korean specialties, and ease of eating,
  118

L
Lactose, 26
Lentils, as protein source, 25

Lettuce, in diet, 28
Lieberman, Dr. Harris, 96, 97, 98
Linguine with shrimp sauce, 261
Liquid carbohydrate strategy, for
     stress relief, 235
Lunch, 69–70
   anti–jet lag
      east-to-west, 219, 223–24
      west-to-east, 209, 214
   avoiding fat traps, 74–76
   brain-powering strategies, 70–72
   effect of eating breakfast on, 60–61
   at ethnic restaurants, 76–78
   at health food restaurants, 78, 80
   of last resort, 79
   preperformance, 129–36
   recommended amounts, 109
   suggested menus, 72–73
Lunch test
   for carbohydrate, 42
   for protein, 41

M

Main dish salads, for lunch, 159
Manhattan-style chowder, 75
Mayonnaise, 75
Melatonin, 90
Mental alertness
   and caffeine consumption, 95–106,
      125, 178–80
   and calorie consumption, 110
Menus
   all-day nibble plan for stress reduc-
      tion, 243–45
   for all-night
      motivated worker dinner, 205
      motivated worker snacks, 205–6
      obligated worker dinner, 196–97
      obligated worker snacks, 197–98
   for at-home preperformance dinner,
      137–38
   for bedtime snacks, 91–92
   for breakfast, 62–63, 130–31
   for conference A.M. coffee breaks,
      182
   for conference afternoon coffee
      breaks, 184
   for conference breakfasts, 150, 182
   for conference dinners, 184–85

   for conference lunches, 156, 160–
      61, 183
   for day after all-night work
      motivated worker breakfast, 206
      obligated worker breakfast, 206
   for dinner, 87–89
   for lunch, 73–74, 131
   for midafternoon snacks, 83–84
   for midmorning snacks, 69
   for predinner snacks, 139
   for preperformance breakfasts, 124–
      25
Mexican food
   for lunch, 74–75
   for conference dinners, 167
Midafternoon, caffeine consumption
   in, 99–100
Midafternoon snacks
   for carbohydrate cravers, 83–84
   need for, 80–81
Midafternoon snack test
   for carbohydrate, 48
   for protein, 47
Midmorning hunger, 61
Midmorning power snacking, 67–69
   in place of breakfast, 59–60
   suggested menus, 61, 69
Midmorning snack test
   for carbohydrate, 46
   for protein, 45
Milk/milk products
   as protein source, 25, 26
   as stimulating, 91
Mind, effect of food on. *See* Food/
   mind/mood responses; Food/
   mind/mood strategies
Minerals, need for, 8–9
Mood, effect of food on. *See* Food/
   mind/mood responses; Food/
   mind/mood strategies
Mornay sauce, 77
Morning performance level,
   role of caffeine in, 98–99
Motivated night worker
   beat-the-clock food plan for, 205–6
   day after breakfast, 206
   food strategies for, 198–204
   morning-after rise-and-shine strate-
      gies, 204
   versus obligated night worker, 189–
      90

Moussaka, 132

N

Nap, need for, to combat jet lag, 224–25
Nervous-eating syndrome, 133–34, 140
Neurotransmitters, 18–19
Neutral foods, 136
Newborn babies, carbohydrates in diet, 248
Night workers
  motivated
    beat-the-clock food plan for, 205–6
    day-after breakfast, 206
    food strategies for, 198–204
    morning-after rise-and-shine strategies, 204
  obligated
    beat-the-clock food plan for all-night mental work, 196–98
    damage limitation techniques for morning after, 195–96
    day-after breakfast, 198
    eating for successful late-night work marathon, 192–95
    food strategies for, 190–91
  obligated versus motivated, 189–90
Noncaffeinated beverages, 178–80
Norepinephrine
  as alertness chemical, 18–19, 20, 58, 86, 141, 204
  as mood-modifying chemical, 13
  production of, 22, 30, 31
  role of caffeine on manufacture of, 98
  strategy for increasing, 31, 71, 116
Nouvelle cuisine, 77
Nutra-Sweet, avoiding foods with, on test days, 37
Nutrition, and food/mind/mood strategies, 8–9
Nutritional counseling, 17–18, 247–49

O

Obligated night worker
  beat-the-clock food plan for all-night mental work, 196–98
  damage limitation techniques for morning after, 195–96
  day-after breakfast, 198
  eating for successful late-night work marathon, 192–95
  food strategies for, 190–91
  versus motivated night worker, 189–90
Oil and vinegar dressing, 79
Oral gratification, need for, and all-day stress, 241–42
Organ meats, as protein source, 26

P

Paper-and-pencil tests, for testing relation of caffeine to mental processes, 97
Pasta, 77
Pasta with seafood and mushroom sauce, 259
Pâté, 115
Peanut butter, for lunch, 78
Peas
  as appetizer, 115
  as protein source, 25
Pork, as protein source, 26
Postperformance relaxers, 141–43
Potato salad, 261
Power eating, 36, 55–93
  and calories, 62
Pregnancy, and caffeine consumption, 104
Premenstrual syndrome, diet management of, 248–49
Preperformance meals, 121–22
  alcohol consumption at, 122
  caffeine consumption at, 122, 125, 126, 127, 135, 140
  for early afternoon performance, 129–34
  for evening performance, 136–41
  for late afternoon performance, 134–36
  lunch
    catered, 132–33
    for early afternoon performance, 129–34
    and eating breakfast, 129–31
    for the late afternoon performance, 134–36

Preperformance meals *(cont.)*
    and the nervous syndrome, 133–34
    ordering of, 131
  for morning performance, 123–29
  principle for, 122
  and sleep induction, 141–43
  timing of, 122–23
Protein, 19–20
  and the alertness effect, 20
  amount needed, 29–30
  at conference breaks, 176–77
  eating before carbohydrate, 113–17
  eating in combination with carbohydrates, 22
  effect of, on serotonin production, 86, 91
  foods with, 24–26
  need for, in lunch, 71
  starting meals with, 175–76
  testing your food/mind/mood response to, 39, 41, 43, 45, 47

R

Reaction-time tests
  for food/mind/mood response, 34–35
  for effect of caffeine on mental processes, 96–97
Recipes, sample, 255–63
Restaurants
  breakfast at, 65, 151–52
  lunch at, 158–61
Restorative snacks, for carbohydrate cravers, 81–83, 128
Roast London broil, 258–59

S

Salad plus, for lunch, 79
Salad/Salad dressing, 75, 76, 115
Sandwiches, for lunch, 159
Seafood Newburg, 132
Seafoods
  for appetizers, 115–16
  for business meals, 76, 77
  for conference dinners, 167
  and ease of eating, 117
Seasonal affective disorder (SAD), diet management of, 249

Serotonin, 13
  as calming chemical, 23, 58, 86, 90, 113, 200, 202, 239
  effect of protein on production of, 71, 86, 91
  as indoleamine, 18
  and the need for insulin, 22, 26, 28, 116, 176–77
  production of, 28, 71, 82, 100, 116
  and sleep induction, 90, 191, 225
Shellfish, as protein source, 25
Simple carbohydrates, 26
Sleep induction
  and choice of bedtime snacks, 90–92
  and choice of dinner meal, 84–86, 88–89
  at conferences, 170
  following performance, 141–43
Snacks
  for the all-night
    motivated worker, 202–3
    obligated worker, 193–94, 197–98
  bedtime, 49, 50, 90–92, 142, 170, 216–17, 226–27
  midafternoon, 83–84
  midmorning, 67–69
  preperformance, 135–36, 138–39
  restorative, 81–83, 128
  and stress management, 241–42, 243–45
Soybean-based foods, as protein source, 25
Spinach, in diet, 28
Spring, Dr. Bonnie, 107
Starches, 27–28
State of mind, importance of, for night workers, 190
Stay-at-homes, breakfast for, 65–67
Stress management, 229–30
  all-day eating plan, 240–42
  all-day nibble plan, 243–45
  carbohydrate "cure" for acute temporary, 231–37
  carbohydrate snacks for, 232, 251–54
  carbohydrates for easing all-day stress, 238–45
  liquid carbohydrate strategy, 234, 235
  morning-to-midnight stress-easing strategy, 242–43

priming the calmness pump, 238
proper "dosage," 232–34
setting scene for relaxation, 236–37
taking time to eat, 234–35
for visceral types, 234
Stroke, link of fat to, 29
Stuffed cabbage roast, 257–58
Sucrose, 26, 27
Sugar, 26, 27
Synchronization, 59

T

Taboullah, 80
Taco chips, 75
Tea. *See also* Caffeine
as source of caffeine, 103
Timing, of preperformance meals,
122–23
Tofu, as protein source, 25
Tortillas, 74–75
Traveling, anti–jet lag tactics for, 207–27
Tryptophan
and albumin in the blood, 22–23
blockage of supply, 31, 115, 177
and the calming effect, 21–23, 113, 202
harm of taking bottled, 23
and the need for insulin, 26, 28
and production of serotonin, 20, 22, 30
supply of, in the all-protein diet, 21
Tyrosine
and the alertness effect, 20, 25

amount needed to produce do-
pamine/norepinephrine, 30
effects of taking excessive amounts
of concentrated, 23
as ingredient in dopamine and norepinephrine, 20, 22, 30, 116, 204

V

Veal, as protein source, 25
Vegetables
for appetizers, 139–40
for lunch, 132, 159–60
Vigilance tests
for effects of caffeine on mental
processes, 97–98
for food/mind/mood response, 34–35
Visceral stress, relief from, 233, 234
Vitamins, need for, 8–9
Vitello tonnato, 256–57

W

White bean soup, 260
Wine. *See also* Alcohol
with dinner, 88, 118–19
Working meals. *See* Business meals

Y

Yogurt
drinking, 67
as protein source, 25, 26